ANCESTRAL WISDOM FOR MODERN HEALING

TRACY HOULE, RHN

CONTENTS

Introduction   v

1. The Hidden Addiction   1
2. The Problem with Going Meatless   13
3. The Power of Local   27
4. Environmental Sabotage   40
5. In the Mood   53
6. Reconnect with Our Ancestors   65
7. You Are What You Eat   79
8. The Case for Boredom   90
9. Collective Food   102
10. All in Your Head   115

Afterword   127
Notes   133
Bibliography   143
About the Author   149
Acknowledgments   151

INTRODUCTION

If you visualize Italy as a heeled boot, Castrignano de' Greci is close to the very tip of the stiletto. It is a relatively isolated village with stone streets winding through a dozen buildings featuring stately brick façades, arched porticos, and iron railings. Outside the village is farmland only occasionally dotted with the *masserie*, the fortified centres of feudal farms that go back centuries, and *Trulli*, the traditional stone huts. Some of the most beautiful beaches in the world stretch along the southern Adriatic coast, whitewashed by the Mediterranean sun. The town was once occupied by Greeks, so even the language spoken there sets them apart—a Greek-influenced dialect of Italian known as Griko. The local culture in Puglia has deep roots, and the region is known for its centuries-old agricultural practices.

This was the childhood home of my grandmother.

My grandmother was born in 1930 to a poor rural family. They sometimes went without food, so she had to take matters into her own hands, picking dandelions and stealing from the edges of farms. I often imagine her as a young girl, her long dark braids trailing behind her as she ran among the dandelion plants that stretched across that landscape, with their broad leaves soaking up the sun and their roots anchored in the rich red soil. She had a wise and deeply rooted intuition, so she knew that the dandelion leaves would sustain her. She wouldn't have described this simple green weed as we would today, a nutritional powerhouse rich in essential vitamins and liver-supportive molecules, but she knew how they would renew her energy and sustain her. Simply, she knew they were good to eat. I imagine her plucking the tall greens and dashing off down the street.

Ancestral Wisdom in Modern Times

Later, when my mother was a child, they lived in a small apartment. No matter what kind of strain they were under financially from time to time, my grandmother ensured the family ate well. She knew how vital real, good food was to a happy and healthy life. In many ways, the way she grew up was to her advantage—she has never eaten or craved fast food because she was never surrounded by it as a child. For her, the "poor man's foods" were what we would today call superfoods. She didn't eat "farm to table" as much as "farm to mouth," and it gave her a life-long understanding of how best to eat.

My mom would reminisce to me about my grandmother peeling off leaves of romaine lettuce and passing them to her, insisting that the "milk was good for her."

My grandmother didn't know that the milky-white substance that seems to bleed from the core of lettuce leaves is called lactucarium. The root of the word lactucarium stems from the Latin *lactus*, meaning *milk* in

English, but of course, it doesn't taste like milk at all. It's slightly bitter and earthy, but fresh tasting. And of course, it is good for you (when consumed in the amounts provided by a healthy serving of lettuce). It helps prevent inflammation and has a calming effect on the nerves, aiding both digestion and sleep.

My grandmother didn't know any of that in scientific terms. But she still knew it. She knew it from her traditional, ancestral ways of eating off the land. Generations of learning passed down—what was poisonous and what was nutritious, what could grow in each season, and how different plants would make you feel.

My grandmother's eating habits may have been partly brought about by need, but in that state, she ate instinctively and treasured the foods that sustained her. She ate, by necessity, according to the seasons. She moved often throughout the day, but her lifestyle would have been considered languid and slow-paced by today's productivity standards.

We've fallen away from that way of life, away from the connection with nature that was passed down to us over hundreds of generations. That's why I wrote this book.

Evolution, by its nature, takes a long time.

For thousands of generations, our genetic ancestors lived as hunter-gatherers and evolved to adapt to different regions as the earliest forms of man expanded across the world. Those genetic adaptations were driven by the need to sustain ourselves with what was available from the environment as efficiently as possible since daily life was active and difficult.

The inception of the human genus, homo, was approximately 2.4 million years ago.[1] Previously,

Australopithecus (like the famous "Lucy" whose fossilized remains were found in Ethiopia) developed only a few of the traits we associate with humanity, like walking on two legs and an omnivorous diet.[2] They had large jaws and flat molars adapted for grinding tough plant fibres. Australopithecus had small brains ranging from about 400 to 550 cubic centimetres.[3]

The separation of the genus homo from Australopithecus is closely linked to a shift in evolutionary trajectory where our ancestors transitioned from primarily foraging and eating small animals to incorporating large amounts of meat into their diets.[4] This transition opened a whole new source of energy, protein, and essential nutrients and provided the raw materials necessary for the evolution of larger, more complex brains. The high-quality protein and fatty acids found in meat enable cognitive abilities crucial for survival, such as problem-solving, social cooperation, and toolmaking.[5] Over time, this co-evolutionary relationship between meat consumption and brain size laid the foundation for the remarkable cognitive abilities that distinguish humans from other primates.

Because meat was the easiest food to get those calories and nutrients from, we continued to evolve as meat-eaters. That meant our brains were not the only physical change we experienced as a species; our guts also developed to support a meat-centred diet. One adaptation of early man was a reduced size of the cecum, a pouch-like structure at the beginning of the large intestine, which is typically larger in herbivores for the fermentation of plant material. Additionally, the small intestine lengthened, giving humans an enhanced capacity for absorbing nutrients from a diet rich in animal proteins and fats. We also developed a higher production of proteases, enzymes that break down proteins, to facilitate the digestion of meat for maximal absorption of necessary nutrients like vitamins A, D, E, K, B6 and B12 as well as essential minerals like calcium, sodium, potassium, iron, and zinc.[6]

While exact timelines are hard to determine, it's evident that these developments took many, many generations to achieve, gradually leading to the complex, intelligent and social animal that we recognize and celebrate as humanity. These genetic adaptations were hard-won over millenniums, allowing man to spread over the world and develop civilization.

And then things began to move a bit faster.

Full-Speed Ahead into Modern Life

Between twelve and ten thousand years ago, about 350 generations ago, humanity began to shift from loose, nomadic family groups to larger tribes.[7] They developed the cultivation of agriculture, both with the farming of grains and legumes and through the domestication of animals and the raising of livestock. During this time, the human diet was still heavily reliant on meat, but it started a major shift toward incorporating plant-based foods on a daily basis.

This change did result in some evolutionary changes, and we can still see the incompleteness of these changes today. Our ancestors' genomes adapted to digesting these new food sources, developing a broader range of enzymes to break down our more varied diets. Genetic mutations related to lactose tolerance, for example, emerged in populations that practised dairy farming, allowing adults to continue digesting lactose beyond infancy. However, as we can see today, these evolutionary changes were not universal, which is why many modern populations struggle with lactose intolerance, despite dairy's prevalence in most modern diets.

These partial adaptations were largely regional. For example, populations with a long history of rice farming have developed genetic adaptations related to starch digestion, while Inuit populations have genetic variations that allow them to efficiently metabolize a high-fat diet typical of their traditional Arctic foods.

But soon, modernity would negate these regional differences in our digestive abilities, establishing populations all over the world with diets that work against even those most recent evolutionary adaptations.

Around six thousand years ago, human civilization began to develop around the world, usually around those mighty rivers that still run through our society centres today: the Amazon, the Nile, the Mississippi, the Indus and the Yangtze. Even more than before, grains and grasses became more and more of a staple in diets, with volume becoming a greater concern than quality of nutrition as population centres exploded and began to double.

Alongside the amazing achievements of these ancient civilizations, we also began to see the origins of inequality in societies. Poor and working-class groups grew larger and larger, and high-volume grains became an affordable way to feed the masses. Meanwhile, the relatively small higher-class populations continued to centre their diets on meats. This pattern was not uniform across civilizations, but it was a general trend that we can still see reflected in modern-day inequalities within and between societies and cultures.

We can even see this trend reflected in modern

language. We use the French-derived "beef" to describe the meat we eat and "cow" to describe the living animal because, after the Norman Conquest of 1066, the English-speaking Saxon peasants could no longer afford to eat their own livestock.[8] So the cow became beef when it was sold to the French-speaking rulers of the country, and that linguistic divide gave us the modern distinction we make today.

Between two hundred and a hundred and fifty years ago, about seven generations, the Industrial Revolution once again brought about a profound change in the way humans eat and live in an even more condensed timeline.

The invention of agricultural machinery, such as the seed drill and the mechanical reaper, increased the efficiency of farming practices, leading to higher yields and reduced labour requirements. However, such degrees of plowing disturbed the soil structure and the complex microbiome it supports. Plowing can alter the availability of nutrients in soil by exposing previously buried organic matter to microbial decomposition and mineralization. This can lead to fluctuations in nutrient levels, which in turn impacts how much nutrients we can derive from our food and the health of our internal gut biome.

Under the influence of the British Empire, farming cultures in Western Europe, the Americas, and India trended toward central consolidation, with larger, more productive farms supporting the communities around them. This allowed for the continued growth of these communities, but it also created a larger disconnect between people and the sources of their own nutrition. Relatively quickly after this shift, these large farms began to focus more on cultivating cash crops like wheat, corn, and cotton, rather than diversified subsistence farming.

This continued the general trend of the masses being relegated to high-volume grains as their primary staple, with the industrial elite having a more diverse and meat-centric diet.

On the very heels of the Industrial Revolution came the so-called "green revolution" and the rapid globalization of food markets. The "green revolution" introduced the development of both specialized high-yield crops and synthetic fertilizers and pesticides. This further allowed for population growth and, in some ways, a more diverse diet for people around the world. However, as I mentioned above, that globalized food market did not account for the subtle regional differences in our digestive abilities. The introduction of pesticides accelerated agriculture's devastating effect on the microbiome of the soil and our waterways.

In the post-World War II era, this trend accelerated across the globe, resulting in the proliferation of fast-food chains and the widespread availability of highly processed, calorie-dense foods. This era also marks a growing inequality between industrialized nations and developing nations, and this gap can again be measured in the differences in our diets. Industrialized nations enjoy all the benefits possible of the globalized food market while profiting from sending cheap, high-volume grains all around the world. Developing nations face a shrinking of their dietary opportunities, as these grains become the vast majority of their diets because of economic need.

And in living memory, the digital revolution has ushered in yet another new age. This age has even more greatly reduced our need to *move* in order to live, with a rapid increase in people living sedentary lifestyles.

It has also created unprecedented access to information, including information about nutrition and health. Many of us turn to this wealth of information about nutrition and agricultural practices to make more informed decisions about our diets and lifestyles.

But among all this information is also a lot of noise. Misinformation, misleading information, and profit-driven "information," create massive confusion around eating, exercise, and lifestyle. People turning to this boundless wealth of knowledge don't find clear advice on how to live healthier, longer, happier lives. They find a quagmire of contradictions.

Many people follow this path to discover some uncomfortable truths about modern animal farming, namely the development of CAFOs. CAFOs, or Concentrated Animal Feeding Operations, are large-scale industrial facilities where animals are raised in confined spaces, for meat, egg, or dairy production. These "farms" hold a large number of animals in relatively small areas, often resulting in environmental and health concerns due to poor waste management and air and water pollution. CAFOs are unquestionably wrong. As a natural reaction to this problem, so many in our society turn to vegetarianism or veganism. However, from an evolutionary diet perspective that I will explore in more detail in this book, this may not be the best choice we can make for our own individual, societal, or planetary health.

In order to make the best decisions for our diets and lifestyles, we need to have a clear understanding of how we got here as a species.

- Developing into highly- active, large-brained meat-eaters: Thousands of generations.

- Developing stationary communities around agriculture: Three hundred and fifty generations.
- The Industrial Revolution: Seven generations.
- The Digital Revolution: Two generations.[9]

Our lifestyles are now changing so rapidly that the mechanics of evolution simply cannot keep up. They have all pointed to massive systemic reductions in the amount of physical activity and work required by humans, especially those living in the developed world.

Our bodies are still essentially the same as those highly active, large-brained meat-eaters that evolution developed over thousands of generations.

This has created an unsustainable gap between what our bodies have developed to eat and do and the way so many of us live our lives. The result of this gap is a rapid increase in physical disability and disease. From an evolutionary perspective, modern metabolic diseases, like chronic fatigue, diabetes, heart disease, and cancer, did not exist prior to the modern era.[10] Some argue that with historical life expectancies, we did not live long enough for these diseases to develop. However, we know by looking at healthy elderly people that these are not diseases of aging, but diseases of modern lifestyle.

In addition, today's children are increasingly being diagnosed with what we once thought of as diseases of the elderly. This increase in ill-health and disease is a symptom of the counter-evolutionary lifestyle and diet that has spread alongside the globalization of the modern world.

Throughout the development of our society, there

continues this trend of separating people from the instinctive, natural way of eating and living that developed in our ancestors and was gently continuing to evolve before the Industrial Revolution led us to fall away from that connection to our own sustenance. In order to bridge the gap between the evolution of our bodies and the evolution of our society, we must have an intentional shift and relearn how to use our intuition - like my grandmother did, to bring us back to eating whole, seasonal foods that our bodies can digest with the highest efficiency.

Where We are Now

When it comes to health and the caretaking of your own body, there are many individual factors and considerations—everything from allergies to your gut biome to regional, cultural, and religious contexts. Many sources of advice on how to optimize your diet and lifestyle for health overflow with judgment and implicit criticisms of how our bodies look. We are shamed for making particular choices and mocked for others.

That is not at all the intention of this book.

Your healthiest body is not about the way you look, but about the way you feel.

So many of my clients come to me frustrated because they consider their diet healthy, at least relatively so, but still, so much of the time, they *just don't feel well*. There is a gap between their impression of what a healthy lifestyle is and the lifestyle that will make them feel the way they want to—strong, healthy, and stable. They are frustrated by so many things: the contradictory advice they've heard, the constant effort to eat better with no real results, and the nagging feeling of sluggishness and discomfort that surrounds them every day. These feelings are an enormous source of unhappiness and poor mental health.

This book will explore the issues with today's eating industry and the natural, ancestral culture it holds hostage. We will examine the ways so many modern foods go against the optimization of our digestion and how to shift your mindset to eat for your own best health. I hope that in reading this book your curiosity is piqued and you become open to trying a path to a new relationship with food, your body, and your intuition.

1

THE HIDDEN ADDICTION

MANY OF US are trapped in a troubled relationship with food.

If you're not sure whether that describes you, ask yourself this. How often do you go to the pantry without a real purpose? You're not hungry, exactly. You've just got that itch for just a little something.

Perhaps you just opened an email that put you in a sour mood, or you feel foggy from an early morning meeting, or it's three p.m., and you've hit your afternoon slump. You may decide you just need a Coke. Or one of the Twizzlers in the bottom drawer of your desk. That last mini donut from that too-early morning meeting. A handful of pepperonis from the fridge. A little treat.

Most of us don't give it any more thought than that, because it feels like a simple fix. There's an uncomfortable little *lack,* and it takes no time at all to fill it. We get our drink and our snack, and very soon, we feel better. The itch is scratched. We are soothed, calmer, and we feel just a little happier.

What could be wrong with that?

The problem is that the itch comes back. And when it does, it's stronger. We need a bit more to feel better. Eventually, the little something we used to enjoy doesn't even feel like a treat. It's just what we need to make that discomfort go away. To get that burst of joy, we need more. And more. And more.

That kind of eating isn't nutrition.

It's addiction.

To understand how trapped we can be by our relationship with food, we have to first step back and examine the bigger picture of how we got here.

The Evolution of Our Diets

Evolution is a slow process, particularly compared to the rapid revolutions of the past one hundred years, and we as a species have not developed the genetic ability to adapt to the level of processed grain and sugar that are so central to modern diets across the world.

Our bodies simply are not built for it.

In the introduction, I touched on how the wheels of history have led to the massive expansion of grains and sugars in our diets. The rate at which this has increased over the last seventy to a hundred years is astounding.

In his article "Cereal Grains: Humanity's Double-Edged Sword," Loren Cordain breaks down the huge disconnect between modern farming and the nutritional needs of our world's population.[1] We consume a remarkably limited number of the thousands of edible plant species that exist in nature, with about seventeen plant species providing 90 percent of the plant-based food supply. Of those farmed plants, only four cereal grains, wheat, maize (corn), rice, and barley, make up more of the world's food supply than the rest of those plant species combined.[2] Cereal grains account for 56 percent of the total calories and 50 percent of the protein consumed on earth.[3]

Grains have become the bedrock of sustaining humanity, despite how ill-suited our bodies are to such a diet.

To start, cereal grains contain no vitamin C, B12, or beta-carotene. Beta-carotene is a precursor to vitamin A, meaning that the body can convert it into active vitamin A as needed. Vitamin A is crucial for various aspects of health, including good vision, a strong immune system, healthy skin and mucous membranes, reproduction and fetal development, and the prevention of cell damage from free radicals.

Cereal grains are also deficient in minerals compared to meat or other plant-based foods, particularly sodium and calcium, which are necessary for fluid balance, nerve function, muscle contraction, and bone health. Furthermore, the minerals grains *do* have in sufficient quantities are often removed through processing before they are consumed. Iron, zinc, magnesium, and manganese can be found in most cereal grains, but are nearly completely removed when grain and rice are processed into white flour and white rice. Yet these very highly processed forms of grains are also the most commonly consumed, especially in the developing world.

This excessive focus on grains isn't just unhealthy; it continues the pattern of inequality in diets that began alongside central agriculture. The most crucial shortcomings of vitamin deficiency in grains are not as acutely felt in Western, industrialized countries as they are in other parts of the world, as Western diets attempt to bridge nutritional gaps through meat consumption and a more varied diet. In developing countries, where cereal grain consumption can make up as much as 80 percent of the calories consumed, nutritional deficiencies and associated illnesses are common.

The most serious consequences of these deficiencies are felt by children. Vitamin A deficiency alone, which increases the severity and mortality of virtually all infectious disease, is estimated to affect twenty to forty million children worldwide.[4]

Our global reliance on these foods is dangerous.

It's also self-perpetuating.

The problem of overreliance on grains is compounded by the fact that sugar and simple starches are highly addictive. Of course, unlike substances such as alcohol, opioids, synthetic stimulants, and other drugs, humans need to eat to survive, leading some to resist applying the word "addiction" to food.

Unfortunately, this resistance stands in the way of understanding how food affects our minds and bodies in ways that are very similar to substances we widely recognize as harmful and dangerous.

When we consume sugar, it activates the brain's release of dopamine, a neurotransmitter associated with pleasure and reward.[5] Over time, repeated exposure to high levels of sugar can lead to desensitization of the brain's reward pathways, requiring even more sugar to achieve the same level of pleasure.[6] We build a tolerance to sugar in the same way users of mood-altering drugs build a tolerance to their forms of self-medication.

What gets you "high" today will only take the edge off tomorrow.

This cycle of consumption followed by immediate

reward followed by more and more need and more (and therefore more consumption) is the cornerstone of what we mean when we say "addiction."

And sugar isn't the only culprit. Dairy and wheat also contain substances with addictive properties. Dairy contains casomorphin, a peptide opioid produced from the digestion of casein, a milk protein.[7] This peptide is formed when enzymes in the stomach break down the casein molecule into smaller pieces. One of these pieces is called an amino acid, and one particular amino acid, glutamic acid, can be converted into casomorphin. This gives dairy its addictive properties.

Gliadomorphin, similarly, is a morphine-like compound that is created during the milling of wheat.[8] The milling process separates the endosperm from the bran and the germ of the wheat kernel. The endosperm is ground into flour, and the bran and germ are used as ingredients in other foods. Gliadomorphin is created when the endosperm is ground into flour.

Both casomorphin and gliadomorphin bind to the same receptors in the brain as their powerful opioid cousins like morphine and heroin.[9] We can also register similar, though of course much milder, changes in mood. Many people experience a calming, sedative effect or a sensuous pleasure when eating these foods because of the interactions of these compounds with their neural receptors.

We even train our brains to expect these compounds when our favourite cheeses and breads touch our tongues, giving us that immediate sense of relief and pleasure. That pattern of expectation: relief, pleasure, and more expectations are the reasons people struggle just as much to change their diets as they do to quit smoking, drink less alcohol, or stop using other self-soothing medications.

That is not to say we should avoid *all* forms of sugar, dairy, and grains with the absolute diligence that we should avoid *all* forms of cocaine and other drastically harmful and addictive substances, but if we can consider addiction a *spectrum* rather than an addictive/nonaddictive binary, we can see a clear parallel that will help us understand our relationship with the foods we crave.

When we feel down, many of us can relate to relying on food to bring us back up. *But not just any food*: we want cookies, ice cream, pizza, or pasta. Or perhaps your particular poison is highly processed fats (the kind found in most fast food), which studies show have the same dopamine reaction and learned tolerance as sugar.

We casually apply the term *craving* to this desire without considering the *compulsion* conveyed by that language. Some foods *just make us feel desperate*.

We can recognize the feelings of physical *need* when we haven't had a "fix" of such foods in a while. We may become lethargic, lightheaded, moody, irritable, or even angry: all those unwanted feelings and symptoms that we learn to suppress by reaching for another donut or chocolate truffle or fried mozzarella stick. I know these feelings all too well.

It is easy to conflate these feelings with hunger but to understand our relationship with these kinds of foods, we must call this reaction what it really is: withdrawal.

Corporate Complicity

Putting people through the continual cycle of craving and withdrawal is also extraordinarily profitable in our corporate-driven world.

Along the way, as the expansion of civilization led to the industrialization and proliferation of corporate production, what began as a convenient way to feed the masses quickly gave way to a deliberate strategy to create and market foods specifically designed to trigger cravings rather than deliver long-lasting nourishment.

In the book *Salt, Sugar, Fat: How the Food Giants Hooked Us,* Michael Moss explains how "Big Food Inc." was successful in getting the public addicted to unhealthy ingredients, and how the industry is built to deliver maximum food addiction and minimum nutrition.[10]

This was not a well-meaning mistake, but a deliberate decision made by major food companies to prioritize sales and growth volume over the health of the communities they serve.

Moss relates how, when challenged to consider how companies may need to hold themselves accountable over growing health concerns, the CEO of General Mills forcefully argued that the company must consider their responsibility to their shareholders. He held up some of the alternate products that are available to people concerned about high fat or sugar content, and then delivered the "bottom line." From the company's perspective, "There's no way we could start down-formulating the usage of salt, sugar, fat if the end result is going to be something that people do not want to eat."[11]

And it is true that without these addiction-triggering ingredients, processed food is not something anyone would want to eat. In an interview with National Public Radio (NPR), Moss describes attempting to eat the processed products without added salt and fat as a "god-awful experience," from straw-flavoured waffles to cereals with metallic aftertastes.[12]

A great deal of money has been invested in cracking the formula of making this food not only tolerable, but irresistible. This goal is called the "bliss point."[13] The bliss point concept involves finding the perfect balance of sweetness from sugar, richness from fat, and savoury flavour from salt to create a taste sensation that is engineered to maximize pleasure so much that consumers are completely hooked on their products.

They call this process, gaining "brand loyalty."[14]

Food scientists and researchers have conducted sensory studies, taste tests, and consumer preference surveys to understand how different combinations of these ingredients affect the taste, texture, and overall appeal of food products. They also will prioritize shelf-stability, consistency, and cost-effectiveness. Research by these industrial companies in nutrition is often perfunctory at best, or entirely ignored.

When food is so greatly divorced from its natural state, the only way companies can get it down the world's throat is to optimize taste and the neural reaction to the food to hook customers on nutritionally empty products.

The strategies they use to do so are indistinguishable from the strategies of alcohol and nicotine companies.

Internally, Coca-Cola does not refer to their best customers as "loyal fans" but as "heavy users."[15] Twenty percent of the people who drink Coke consume 80 percent of the product produced. This statistic is mirrored in the alcohol industry, with 10 percent of users consuming 60 percent of alcohol sold.[16] These heavy users contribute to the high-profit margins of both industries, which both use brand loyalty, social advertising, and targeted marketing to increase their footholds in the market, at the expense of the health of the heavy users that keep those companies afloat.

This addiction trap was built up around us by the growing worldwide reliance on grains and grasses and the corporate-driven greed to create foods based on what people will buy, regardless of nutritional value.

Once we accept that food cravings are a form of withdrawal and understand how the system designed by Big Food does not serve our best interests, we can begin to work our way out of the trap.

But we wouldn't call it an "addiction" if it were easily broken. I have seen many clients struggle, particularly when they try a makeshift, DIY approach to giving up these foods. Getting ourselves off grains and sugar requires a process, guidance, understanding, and support to break the cycle.

When coming off processed carbs (which is what modern grains are) and sugar, we need to give ourselves a few days to gird ourselves for the process. Because, at first, it feels like going through hell. It can be enormously difficult to sit in that discomfort of withdrawal for long enough to pass through it. You may experience fatigue, headaches, mood swings, muscle aches, brain fog, lightheadedness, and digestive discomfort. It may take several attempts, as the temptation to give up is strong, and we are used to giving in to the need to feel better now.

As you might imagine (or as you may have experienced yourself), the process can be very stressful, a result that can have additional effects on your body. Hormones like cortisol and adrenalin, both of which are necessary for survival, regulate the body's response to stress. Dietary changes can influence the production and activity of these hormones, and in turn, stress hormones can also affect dietary behaviours and metabolism, creating another cycle that is incredibly difficult to break. In high levels, stress hormones like cortisol can increase appetite and promote the storage of fat, damage gut health, block the ability to absorb nutrients, and raise blood sugar levels.

Many people habitually combat stress with eating, and this can create a feedback loop between stress and hormone production. We eat to combat stress, which releases stress hormones, which makes us want to eat even more, which gradually makes us feel worse and more stressed.

To complicate this trap even further: some of us have a genetic predisposition to sugar and fat addiction. These genetic variations can influence behaviour and addiction risk in the same way they can with generational alcoholism. This addiction can lead to obesity and cardiovascular issues if the habit is acted on consistently and left untreated.

For example, I have the CT variant for the GLUT2 gene. The GLUT2 gene (also known as SLC2A2) encodes a glucose transporter protein that plays a crucial role in the transport of glucose across cell membranes, particularly in the liver, pancreas, and intestine. Variants of this gene can have a wide range of effects on how our bodies use and process glucose. They can also lead to the development of metabolic disorders, including type 2 diabetes, and the rarer Fanconi-Bickel Syndrome, which impairs glucose and galactose metabolism.

Ultimately, what that means for me is that if I am not careful about my sugar intake, I will continue to crave more and more (and consequently, enjoy small amounts less and less). If I give into the cravings over an extended period of time, I am more likely to develop a metabolic disorder, most commonly type 2 diabetes.

Like all genetic conditions, the condition runs in my family, so we all must be watchful of our sugar intake in order to safeguard our health and well-being.

Having this knowledge about my body and my family's genetic predispositions doesn't make me fearful, but rather empowers me to develop the mindset and practice I need to make the best choices available to me.

Just because the trap is there, doesn't mean we have to stay in it.

A Path for Change

So, considering all we know about addictive foods and the potential consequences of continuing with an unexamined diet, how can we move forward?

Food knowledge is better, by far than any particular diet plan. Having more knowledge about our food allows us to make better choices about what we eat.

Most people already know how hard it is to change the way you eat, how much you move, and your overall lifestyle. Understanding the reasons for this difficulty is a huge step toward conquering it.

In reality, the issue is not just food. An extremely challenging problem we face in modern society is that we live in a time of overwhelming abundance: processed food at our fingertips, the internet and social media in our pockets, and entertainment around the clock. Our precious dopamine reward pathway is constantly on overdrive making it continuously more challenging to enjoy a walk in the park, a sunset, or eating food that doesn't light up our brain to that corporate-serving bliss point.

But once we know what is happening in our brains, we can begin making the choices that will better regulate our needs and cravings, allowing us to derive more pleasure from the things that are wholly and fully good for us. Dramatically reducing consumption of processed food, cereal grains, and addictive foods and replacing them with whole, unprocessed ingredients can have amazing, long-term effects on your health and happiness. It doesn't have to be complicated—in fact, the simpler the better.

In later chapters, we will explore how to establish a diet of whole foods, focus on simplicity, and navigate your way around the many arms of the trap.

Establishing a healthier diet requires time and patience, but breaking that cycle is better in the long run. You can get back to the balance of homeostasis needed to feel well in the long term.

2

THE PROBLEM WITH GOING MEATLESS

IN THE YEARS following World War II, there was a major shift not only in how food was processed and manufactured, but also in how animals were raised for meat. As life returned to a new post-war normal, a booming economy and rising birth rates created unprecedented demand. Farmers responded by abandoning traditional methods in favour of confining animals in increasingly smaller spaces, maximizing the poundage of meat that could be produced by an acre of industrial farmland.

The Rise of Industrial Farming

Chickens were first.

Between 1950 and 1960, the North American production of broiler chickens exploded. To maintain their flocks, farmers began to keep more chickens to a cage, soon stacking cages three or four levels high. This shift in practices also led farms to follow the corporate model—farms that could concentrate their meat production bought out more and more smaller farms by the year.

Through the 1970s and 80s, pork and cattle farms followed suit. In only a few short decades, the way meat was farmed was completely turned on its head. In 1966, one million farms reared fifty-seven million pigs. By 2001, those millions of pigs were raised by eighty thousand farms. The production of broiler chickens increased 1,400 percent in the latter half of the 20th century. At the same time, producers shrank from 1.6 million farms to only twenty-seven thousand.[1]

Concentrating animals in this way created toxic centres of pollution, with the areas around these industrial farms suffering from the strain of waste disposal, ground and surface water pollution, and excess methane production. In 1972, the Clean Water Act defined these meat production centres as "AFOs" (animal feeding operations). By 1976, as the trend toward rearing more and more animals on lesser acreage continued, "CAFO" was added as a distinct term, which was defined as any operation that confined over a thousand "animal units" (a thousand pounds of living animals) for more than forty-five days a year.

These centres can ruin communities, and frequently the communities most at risk are poor, rural areas where land is cheap and money is scarce in the local population. These communities can spend decades trying to fight the effects of proximity to these operations. For example, Uniontown, Alabama is plagued by a massive chicken CAFO and a large catfish farm, both of which have had devastating effects on the Black Warrior River Basin.[2]

The noise and the stench—which is so powerful on its own that it causes increased rates of asthma and bronchitis—from these centres is the least of the community's concerns. The chicken facility has attempted to use the enormous amount of fecal waste produced to fertilize surrounding pastures, but this is nowhere near an adequate solution. Any given patch of soil can only absorb so much of the fertilizing minerals. The excess nitrogen and phosphorous end up in the local waterways as run-off, and often into groundwater and subsequently, into the drinking water as well.

Uniontown does not have a mechanical treatment plant and instead relies on a cheaper method of collecting sewage in a lagoon system where solids settle to the bottom and the liquid can be sprayed on a field in the expectation that natural vegetation and microbes can break down the minerals and pathogens in the waste.

The lagoon system's capacity to do this is overwhelmed by the catfish farm alone. This leaves the community scrambling for solutions, but because a large portion of the community is reliant on these operations for their incomes, negotiations between the town and the companies are slow and contested. In the meantime, the waterways nearby become more and more polluted.

Mass-Produced Meat is Unhealthy Meat

The environmental impact on communities is not the only problem with these operations—the quality of food that comes out of these facilities is drastically inferior to that produced by smaller farms where the animals are not kept in such conditions. The unnatural environment for the animal causes stress, changing the body chemistry of the animal. Animals kept in CAFOs often have impaired immune systems because of this stress, which is exacerbated by how quickly disease and infection spreads in the condensed spaces. In a CAFO, it is impossible to sequester ill animals, so instead the entire stock is given high amounts of antibiotics to reduce animal loss.

Many of these high-volume meat producers will dismiss concerns that the meat from animals raised in such conditions is significantly less healthy to consume. They would have us believe that meat is meat.

However, we can measure one way CAFO-raised meat is inferior through the ratio of Omega 6 to Omega 3 fatty acids. Fatty acids are materials necessary for health and are obtained entirely through diet.

Omega-3 fatty acids are known for their anti-inflammatory properties and are crucial for brain function, heart health, and reducing the risk of chronic diseases such as cardiovascular disease and arthritis. Omega-6 fatty acids are a type of unsaturated fat that is commonly found in vegetable oils, nuts, seeds, and processed foods. The body can use moderate amounts of these fatty acids in cell membrane structure, hormone production, and inflammation regulation. However, excessive consumption of omega-6 fatty acids, especially in relation to omega-3 fatty acids, can cause increased inflammation and chronic disease.

The desired ratios of these acids are somewhat disputed, ranging from an equal one-to-one ratio to a moderate four-to-one ratio.

Meat produced by CAFOs far exceeds these ratios, often as high as forty-to-one.[3]

Animals raised in CAFOs are almost universally fed a diet high in grains, mostly corn and soybeans, which are concentrated in Omega-6 fatty acids, but with quite very little Omega-3. (This also contributes to high Omega-6 levels in processed foods, which are high in grains compared to other vegetable matter.)

Comparatively, grass-fed animals produce meat with a much healthier ratio of Omega 6 to Omega 3 fatty acids. Coen Farms in Alberta, Canada, for example, raises grass-fed, free-range cattle and produces beef with a remarkable two-and-a-half-to-one ratio of fatty acids.

CAFOs are a blight on our environments and produce meat that contributes to ill health.

The Misguided Push for Meatless Diets

Understandably, as the effects of this shift in practice came more to light in the 1970s through the early 00s, so too came the growing popularity of vegetarianism and veganism. This reaction came in part through concern for animal welfare, but also from fears regarding the effects of high-fat diets on health. While this was an understandable reaction, this knee-jerk response to cut out meat completely from diets was and continues to be a misguided choice, especially from the perspective of nutrition.

One immediate impact of going meatless is an increased diet of ultra-processed foods. In a study for the Journal of Nutrition, Josephine Gehring found that higher avoidance of animal-based foods corresponded to an increase in reliance on highly processed foods in their diets, often as high as a third to forty percent of their total consumed calories.[4]

The growing popularity of meatless diets has been met with "innovations" from large food corporations who see this as an opportunity to meet a growing market niche with Vegan-labelled products that, while they cost less to produce, often cost more than their traditional counterparts. They can charge more because the marketing of the vegetarian or vegan label gives the veneer of a healthier, more ethical lifestyle. The halo effect of these companies drives sales and perpetuates the myths that meatless diets are superior.

Corporate Influence of Food Policies

Big Food lobbyists have also had a profound impact on health policy and diets in the West. The guidelines written and designed by our governments are supposed to be easy to follow, and sensible advice on how to eat a healthy diet for most people. However, its creation and revisions over the years have been heavily influenced by lobbyists from corn, sugar, and chemical companies.

Both Canada and the United States have policies that attempt to limit corporate influence on government policy but have not held up to the pressure and influence of Big Food. Lynda Powell, professor of political science at the University of Rochester, demonstrated how profound this influence can be in her book *The Influence of Campaign Contributions in State Legislatures.*[5] The result of this influence can be seen in the gap between what research shows about nutrition and the dietary guidelines and policies put forth by the government.

Part of the web of corporate influence on government policy comes from the revolving door between lobbyists and government agencies. In the US, the Obama administration attempted to clamp down on this practice in 2009, signing an executive order forbidding lobbyists from working for agencies that they had lobbied known as the "cooling off" period. This policy did not stand up for long, and by the time Donald Trump took office, cooling off rules were waived as a matter of routine. One such waiver occurred when the USDA hired Kailee Tkacz to work as adviser to the 2020 revisions of the dietary guidelines. Tkacz accepted the position immediately after lobbying for years for the Corn Refiners Association, which represents the biggest producers of high-fructose corn syrup.[6] It is clear these moves are deliberately aimed at giving access to and influence over government agencies in charge of regulating food industries directly to the industries they are supposed to regulate.

Reactions to animal conditions in CAFOs, the misconceptions about fat and cholesterol that arose in the latter half of the twentieth century, and the influence of the sugar and grain-driven food lobby have all driven the popularity of meatless diets. These trends are also supported by social media campaigns, often tainted by misleading or completely incorrect information about nutrition. As the popularity of this misguided trend grew, so did a number of myths surrounding the healthfulness and success of meatless diets to address these issues.

Myths of the Meatless Diets

Myth 1: "You Can Get All the Nutrients You Need"

The first myth of the meatless diet is that it is easy to consume the necessary protein, fats, vitamins, and minerals on an entirely plant-based diet.

The most crucial term in understanding why this is a myth is bioavailability, which is the proportion of a drug or other substance that enters the circulation when introduced into the body and so is able to have an active effect. In other words, bioavailability is how much a nutrient from the food will actually be absorbed in the body for use after we eat it. This distinction is crucial in understanding both how a food's lab-tested chemical properties can differ from the actual and practical effects on health.

This difference can also contribute to the myths surrounding foods, as many foods are advertised based on their lab-tested properties, which leads people to assume their bodies can actually access and utilize these nutrients. But this isn't always the case. The human body is enormously complicated, with many components affecting how nutrients are absorbed when consumed alone or in conjunction with other substances. Certain forms of iron, for example, such as heme iron found in animal products, are more readily absorbed by the body than non-heme iron found in plant-based foods. Some nutrients work against each other, like how high calcium intake can inhibit the absorption of magnesium and vice versa.

Functional Medicine Practitioner and author Chris Kresser provided this comparison in a 2022 interview. "Let's just take calcium in spinach as an example. You can look at a cup of spinach and say, wow, there's actually quite a bit of calcium in there. But then you realise that spinach also contains phytic acid, which inhibits the absorption of minerals like calcium. And there have been studies that have shown that you need about eight cups of spinach in order to get the same bioavailable amount of calcium that you get from drinking one glass of milk."

As noted in the previous chapter, the increase of grain and sugar consumption correlates with the growing number of nutrient deficiencies around the world. Along with vitamin A, the most common are iron, Vitamin B12, and calcium deficiencies, and these nutrients are absorbed far more efficiently from animal-source foods.

It is not only a few nutrients that are more easily absorbed by animal-sourced foods than plant-based foods, but the majority and most essential of them. The DIAAS of a food refers to the Digestible Indispensable Amino Acid Score, which measures the digestibility and amino acid composition of a protein source. Animal-based proteins universally score higher than plant-based, even when plant-based proteins are isolated and concentrated.

The fact that the nutrients found in plants generally are less available to digestive absorption is likely due to common trends in plant evolution. From an evolutionary perspective, plants don't want to be eaten any more than animals do. Animals evolved several categories of adaptation to avoid being consumed before they can reproduce—evasion, camouflage, poison, defence, or even just a very quick maturation and reproductive rate. These were not options for most plant species.

But plants do have defence mechanisms! Some plants have in fact *anti-nutrients* specifically evolved to make them difficult to digest. Phytic acids, found in seeds and grains, can bind to minerals such as calcium, iron, zinc, and magnesium, reducing their absorption in the digestive tract. Oxalates in foods like spinach and beet greens can bind to calcium (also found in spinach) to form insoluble crystals. Lectins, in grains and nightshades, can bind to carbohydrates and prevent their absorption. They can also cause inflammation in the gut and digestive issues, passing food too quickly through the body to be digested fully and utilized.

For the plant, this ensures that seeds survive the

passage through the digestive system and the plant species continue into further generations.

Fermentation can break down anti-nutrients so they can be absorbed more easily. Vegetarian animal species adapted the ability to do this along their digestive tracts. Humans, however, did not evolve this way, which makes it very difficult to get the essential nutrients for our bodies to function as fully intended on a plant-based diet.

Myth 2: "Meat Raises Your Cholesterol"

The second myth surrounding meatless diets is that one can prevent heart disease, type 2 diabetes, or cancer with a plant-based diet. These diseases are metabolic in nature, driven by lifestyle and environment more than genetics.

Through the late fifties to the early seventies, the leading trends of popular health science, driven primarily by the research of Ancel Keys, blamed high-fat diets and cholesterol as the primary causes of heart and coronary disease. This presumption quickly led to the proliferation of manufacturers promoting low-fat or no-fat versions of their products. It also contributed to the growing popularity of meatless diets, as cutting meat was seen as the simplest and most direct way to cut out fats.

However, more recent research has largely debunked this hypothesis. First, it was discovered that cholesterol is not all created equal. Health professionals recognize that high-density lipoprotein (HDL) cholesterol is "good" because it helps remove cholesterol from the bloodstream. It has also become clear that the size and density of low-density lipoprotein (LDL) particles, as well as other factors such as inflammation and oxidative stress, may play a more significant role in heart disease risk than total cholesterol levels alone. Re-examining the early research shows that the correlation between a diet high in saturated fats and heart disease is weak and inconsistent, especially compared to other dietary and lifestyle factors.

The more we learn about metabolic disorders and the bioavailability of nutrients in foods, the more it becomes clear that the overconsumption of processed grains and sugars is the culprit behind this rise in disease, not the consumption of animal protein or fats alone.

Myth 3: "Eating Meat is Bad for the Environment"

The third myth surrounding meatless diets is the assumption that it is the only path toward saving our planet and that eating meat is in itself bad for the environment.

As we explored at the top of this chapter, CAFOs are undeniably bad for their surrounding areas. The meat they produce is also far less healthy than ideal. However, it does not follow that the best and only way we can save or reverse these effects must come at the expense of our own nutrition.

The good news is there is a growing movement that is doing exactly what needs to be done to move back toward planetary and individual health—and it is not cutting out meat. Regenerative farming involves farming to eliminate synthetic fertilizers, pesticides, and other chemicals.

Large-scale mono-agriculture is also contributing to CO^2 in our atmosphere, driving climate change and increasing the global average temperature.

Monoculture farming, which involves growing a single crop species in a given area, has been adopted by farmers because its simplicity seems to allow greater yields.

However, monoculture farming causes significant harms over time. Single-crop fields become easy targets for pests, leading to increased use of pesticides, which in turn contaminate soil and water sources. Second, monoculture depletes soil nutrients, leading to soil degradation and a loss of fertility. Farmers often compensate by using chemical fertilizers, which further harm soil health and local ecosystems.

Monoculture crops lead also to soil erosion and poor water retention, which requires more irrigation and depletes local water sources. The lack of biodiversity in monoculture systems also impacts pollinators like bees, which are crucial for many crops' reproduction. While it initially attracted farmers for its simplicity, monoculture farming comes with a great deal more costs than it does benefits.

Crop rotation, smart fertilizer use, moderated pesticide application, efficient water use, and a shift toward polyculture can help mitigate these negative impacts, promoting a healthier and more resilient agricultural system.[7]

Agriculture has the reputation of being one of the biggest contributors to climate change, but industry and transportation are far more damaging and need to be our priorities in reducing carbon output. In addition, with the proper livestock and poly-agriculture practices, greenhouse gases can be sequestered and the impact negated.[8]

The Power of Regenerative Agriculture

Regenerative agriculture seeks not only to reduce the impact of mono-agriculture and CAFOs, but also to reverse the effects of decades of harmful practices. The primary principles of regenerative agriculture include conservation tillage, crop and grazing rotation, biodiversity, and high caution regarding any application of chemical or added fertilizer.

When we repeatedly plow large plots of land, we are directly contributing to the heating of the earth. It erodes the soil and releases large amounts of carbon dioxide into the atmosphere. Low and no-till methods allow farmers to minimize the physical disturbance of the soil, keeping the soil healthy and increasing the nutrient density of the food grown in that soil.

Farmers began to understand the importance of crop rotation after the devastating effects of the dust bowl, where bad farming practices rendered once valuable pastureland into barren wastes for generations. But traditional contemporary farmers have only learned part of the lesson, often rotating crops the bare minimum to prevent total soil erosion. By including the use of cover crops and rotational grazing in addition to rotating crops, farmers can keep the soil high in beneficial microbial activity and closer to what is found in wild, natural environments, while still producing quality food.

These practices also intentionally raise the quality of the life of the animals in their care and the quality of soil that feeds the microorganisms important for healthy plant food. Healthier animals have repeatedly been shown to produce healthier meat. Because animal protein is the most potent source of bioavailable nutrients for humans, the best path toward *both* planetary and individual health is not cutting out meat from our diets but incorporating these sensible practices broadly across the agricultural industry, whether it's meat or plants being consumed.

As destructive as CAFOs and mono-agriculture can be and as important as reducing their impact on our environment is, eschewing meat as a way to do so is throwing the baby out with the bath water. On the contrary, we have evolved to be meat-eaters, so it is not in our best interest to remove this valuable source of nutrients from our diets. It is crucial that we fight against the use of outdated farming practices and throw our support toward farmers who are using sustainable practices for both our bodies and the health of our planet.

3

THE POWER OF LOCAL

LEARNING to see how many systems are in place that contribute to our ill health can feel overwhelming. But there are ways to take control over your own consumption if you're willing to persist through breaking the habits, fighting through the withdrawal systems, and overcoming the social pressures surrounding food and eating. By making some deliberate, simple changes, we can make a real change to our own health and the environment that sustains us.

One Ingredient at a Time

My personal journey toward taking control of my health through diet started with my son. He was born in 2006, and by the age of six he was plagued by daily stomach and digestive pain. It was heartbreaking to see him suffer every single night. I took him to a doctor, who suggested he was lactose intolerant.

That was the whole of that conversation, which I found enormously frustrating. Although we did eliminate dairy at that time, it didn't stop all the symptoms. Sure, eliminating dairy is a change we should be able to make easily enough, but I didn't understand *why* such a common food would give my child such trouble. The more I thought about it, the more I began to wonder whether my son's symptoms were the only symptoms in our household. I wondered if there was something wrong with other parts of our diets.

I couldn't stand to see my son suffer, but I realised I had become inured to my own discomfort as well. I also often suffered from digestive pain. Was it simply that I was lactose intolerant, too, or was there more to this?

Ever since I was a teenager, I have struggled with hormonal issues and abnormal periods. But around the time my son was being diagnosed lactose intolerant, I also suffered miscarriages.

I was often told that all these symptoms were completely *normal*. But there's a huge difference between *normal* and *common*. Just because something occurs frequently doesn't mean it's the way things should be. Perhaps we didn't just have to accept these symptoms just because they weren't unusual.

I explored naturopathic medicines, but they didn't provide any more of a clear, structured plan than conventional medicine did. One naturopath recommended more protein and supplements but didn't provide any real answers for what was happening in my body or provide the root cause of my symptoms. That's not to say that all doctors or naturopaths aren't valuable, I still use them when I need them. It was just my experience when the root cause was not on their radar or something we discussed, so I was left with more questions.

I continued to search because I wanted to understand,

not only what I should and shouldn't be eating, but *why and how we got here.*

Exploring Ancestral Eating

Through my research, I discovered the Paleo diet. The Paleo diet is the idea of eating in an ancestral way, the way our Paleolithic ancestors ate, focusing on animal proteins and the kinds of produce that would be found and consumed during the era while completely avoiding grains and processed foods.

From there, I looked into what was wrong with eating grains and dairy, turning up, little by little, all the horrifying truths I've covered so far in this book and more.

The Paleo diet opened a door to explore *why* these foods came with these side effects. In terms of fat content and other traditional ways of measuring the health of foods, dairy wasn't so bad. But when I thought in terms of ancestral eating, I began to question if it was really an appropriate food—not just for myself, my son, and others with lactose intolerance—but as a species. In the first two years of life, like all mammals, we consume mostly milk, but unlike any other mammal, we continue to do so in the form of animal milk into adulthood.

The more I read about grains, the more I became convinced that they were also not right for our bodies, especially at the rate we consume them today. So, as an experiment at first, our family adopted a version of the Paleo diet.

At the time, I knew myself well enough to know that if there was junk food in the house, I would eat it. I didn't have the willpower to resist something literally at hand, so I threw away everything that was to be no longer in our diet. We focused on making animal protein central to every meal, including simple one- or two-ingredient vegetable side dishes, and avoiding grains, processed foods, most dairy, legumes, and most sugars.

Our digestive problems were the first to clear up, with both my son and I having easier digestion and no more pain. My daughter was also less bloated. My husband lost weight.

Then, something happened that I never expected. Amazingly, my hormones came into balance for the first time in my adult life. My cycle normalized and became easier and more predictable. Within six months of making this dietary change, I was pregnant.

I never miscarried again.

Seeing how much nutrition could change my life ignited in me a passion for understanding as much as I could about the connection between food and health. I continued to read as much as I could on my own until 2014 when—seven months pregnant with my youngest child—I registered for nutrition school.

I chose the Canadian School of Natural Nutrition for its accessibility and focus on holistic nutritional practices. After two years of studying, I became a nutritionist. By then, I knew that simply gaining the theoretical knowledge and the science behind nutrition was not enough. I wanted to be able to directly help people experience the amazing, life-affirming changes that my own family had experienced.

I went on to the Academy of Culinary Nutrition, where I learned how to teach people to cook healing foods in their very own kitchens, and I gained certification as a Culinary Nutrition Expert. By this time, I was growing to see food as our most essential form of medicine. I wanted to use my newfound understanding to get to the root causes of chronic illness, so I enrolled in a Functional Nutrition program. Finally, I felt I needed to better understand the mental and social barriers between people and their healthiest selves, so I also went on to train in the Institute for the Psychology of Eating. The human body is complicated and affected by diet and our environments in so many ways, I knew I also had to diversify my training to see the problem from as many perspectives as possible. It's been a long but fulfilling journey.

In all my training and my experience helping clients meet their nutritional needs, one consistent takeaway is that while big changes are always hard, we do not have to make them even harder by making them *complicated*.

It is a natural instinct, when making a major lifestyle change, to over-do it in the planning stages and try to implement a lot of stressful regimens all at once. But going from not spending much time reflecting on your diet at all to tracking every single calorie and nutrient is not a sustainable change for most people. It sets people up to fail, which psychologically reinforces both poor self-image and the lifestyle status quo.

The Challenges with Food Security Programs

The challenges of habit, addiction, and social pressures are difficult enough to endure. But it's worth noting that these challenges increase tenfold in the absence of economic stability. Those in the developing world and those without economic mobility must rely on government programs to meet their dietary needs—and those programs are not designed with values in mind.

In the United States, the SNAP program, formerly

known as the Food Stamp Program, dominates as the largest federal nutrition assistance program, serving forty to forty-five million people at any given time, averaging at between 12 – 13 percent of the total population of the United States.[1] Enrolment is not static, as some families and individuals receive benefits for short periods of time while others rely on the program for decades. Eligibility for SNAP is based on factors such as household income, expenses, and the number of people in the household.

What started as part of President Lyndon B. Johnson's war on poverty has ballooned into a massive program, costing tens of billions of dollars per year. SNAP beneficiaries include a range of races and age groups, though vulnerable populations are of course more heavily represented. 36 percent are white, 25 percent are African Americans (this is disproportionate, as African Americans only make up 12 percent of the total population), 17 percent Hispanic, and 4 percent Asian or Native American. Millions are veterans, seniors, or people with mental or physical disabilities. Nearly half are children.[2]

SNAP is continually the centre of both political debate and grandstanding. There is an enormous need for support, so SNAP is a vital anti-poverty and anti-hunger tool, and that is precisely why it desperately needs reform. Examining the US population, we can see that those who are enrolled in SNAP have somewhat better health than those who have the same economic needs but are not enrolled. It's clear that SNAP does provide help; after all, fed is better than unfed. However, it can and must do better.

In a 2017 study at the College of William and Mary, Professor Dr. Zach Conrad found that "individuals participating in SNAP exhibited higher total and cardiovascular disease mortality."[3] While SNAP successfully protects against basic hunger, it is an utter failure at protecting against diet-related diseases and addictions and does not provide its enrollees with the essential nutrients for health and longevity. Those enrolled in the SNAP face higher rates of metabolic illness than those of the greater population because of the systems that make junk calories cheaper and easier to obtain than fresh, quality food.

Rather than providing a path for equity, it continues the millenniums-old trend of disparity of diets between the upper and working classes.

In his book, *The Food Fix: How to Save Our Health, Our Economy, Our Communities, and Our Planet-One Bite at a Time,* Mark Hyman, MD understands how central food is to the health of our global community, both on an individual and societal level.[4] He seeks to connect the dots of how "food is at the nexus of most of our world's health, economic, environmental, climate, social, and even political crises" and why "fixing our food system is central to the health and well-being of our population" and even "the very survival of our species."[5] He explores the impacts of food policy on inequity, disease and the environment, and outlines the myriad issues with programs like SNAP that are heavily influenced by lobbying from Big Food and Big Agriculture.

In a study examining the diets of SNAP participants and nonparticipants: SNAP participants consumed 44 percent more fruit juice, 56 percent more potatoes, and 61 percent more soft drinks.[6] One report calculated that seven billion dollars of food stamps are spent on sugary beverages like sodas each year. 75 percent of the food purchased using SNAP benefits are classified as ultra-processed foods that contain little to no nutrition beyond providing calories. As Hyman puts it, "Thanks to federal support for corn, soy, and grains, junk food is now cheaper than ever (with the help of taxpayers' dollars), and consumers are exposed to a conveyor belt of empty, disease-producing calories."[7]

The problem, however, extends beyond the difference in availability between junk and fresh food. Big Food sees this pool of billions as an opportunity—not to help those most in need—but to increase its profit margins. To take the highest possible advantage of the products with the greatest profitability, corporations directly target low-income SNAP participants with their marketing strategies, selling them their low-nutrition, high-profit processed foods.

A 2018 study of marketing presence in grocery stores found that on the first week of the month, grocery stores and other limited food retailers displayed over four times more advertising for sugar-sweetened beverages like sodas.[8] This was no coincidence, as grocery stores know that these days are when SNAP beneficiaries receive their monthly benefits. Wealthier neighbourhoods didn't see the same increase in junk food ads. This is partly because corporations know that those who are not reliant on assistance are less likely to vary their consumption habits from week to week. Second, it is a deliberate strategy to target those with limited spending power to spend what they have on bliss point designed, heavily manufactured food that represents their greatest profits. The regularity of SNAP benefit dispensation serves them this strategy on a silver platter. The 2018 study suggested that "policy changes, like extending SNAP benefit issuance, may mitigate these effects."[9]

It is obvious that the government cannot dictate the diets of citizens, even those on federally funded food assistance programs. Attempts to do so would not only be a massive governmental overstep; it would also be simply ineffective. However it can and should disrupt Big Food's strategic stranglehold on these funds by reforming the SNAP program to both increase the ease and availability of healthy food to participants and lessen the effects of targeted advertising. Additionally, expanding the subsidies so that local and environmentally sound producers can more easily provide food for those on SNAP benefits would clear the path for positive change for everyone.

Spending Wisely on Nutrition-Dense Food

This is not as challenging as it might seem on its face.

It's an unfortunate cliché that healthier, more nutritionally dense food often costs more by volume. But in balance, that somewhat higher price tag can be offset by deliberate practices that can keep you satiated through fewer dollars.

Five pounds of high-quality ground beef can cost upwards of forty dollars, whereas the same volume of rice can cost as little as four dollars. However, nutritionally, five pounds of beef goes a long way. With three meals centred on animal protein, you'll be satiated for longer with much less volume of food. Five pounds of rice is barely better than starvation, leading to greater feelings of hunger and undernourishment.

If we consider the nutritional benefit rather than the sheer poundage of our food, the cost differences aren't so great.

The real costs of poor eating also include so much

more than the price of the food itself. Feeling sick from bad eating makes it difficult to work well and enjoy time away from work. Chronic illness costs huge amounts of money and time. In the end, the investment is not only worth it, but also a no-brainer.

But thinking this way about food isn't just about limiting our spending. What we spend our money on also reflects our values. Establishing clear values around both what goes in our bodies and where our dollars go is beneficial for us both physically and mentally, and it also helps sustain our local and global environments.

Our ancestors, by necessity, ate seasonally. Meat was available year-round, but vegetable matter varied greatly throughout the year. Depending on the part of the world, fruit was a brief and seasonal treat. We can move closer to replicating this by increasingly buying locally produced food. This in turn also helps smaller farms and allows them to move toward the regenerative practices I described in the previous chapter. Farmers markets can be a good place to start, but it can be sometimes difficult to find organic food and be certain the foods on display are grown under the conditions that are advertised.

Connecting to local farms and buying food directly is the best way to get the very best food and make sure the most of your money is spent toward better practices. Unfortunately, most people don't even know this is an option.

Many communities in the US and Canada have CSAs, or Community Supported Agriculture. CSAs are a unique marketing agreement between the farmer and the consumer. The consumer pays the farmer a fee in advance of the growing season and in return, the farmer provides the consumer a variety of fresh produce every week during the growing season.

Canada and the US also have databases consumers can use to find local growers and connect directly to the farms to order food. In Canada, Regeneration Canada is a nonprofit organization dedicated to promoting soil regeneration in order to mitigate climate change, restore biodiversity, improve water cycles, and support a healthy food system. They provide the public with searchable, trustworthy information about connecting to local farms. In the US, FarmMatch is a very simple and easy-to-use platform for connecting to farms that meet their sustainable practice standards. Users can simply enter their zip codes, choose a farm, and order food.

With a little bit of planning and deliberation, we can access high-quality, value-aligned food without spending more than we can afford. With a little practice, you can even save money, opening possibilities for improving our health, our environment, and the most vulnerable in our global community.

Navigating the Grocery Store

For better or for worse, one of the most immediately visible effects of the globalization of the food industry is the standardization of grocery stores. In nearly any grocery store in the developed world, you can walk in and find, immediately to your right or left, the produce section. These are ubiquitously against the wall and in the corner so the displays can access the water lines for the hydrocoolers most commonly used to keep lettuces and other thirsty vegetables moist (and, consequently, shiny and appealing to shoppers). On the opposite wall are typically the meat and seafood counters. They are situated along a wall to provide the employee areas needed for additional refrigeration, packaging, and (for those lucky enough to still have in-house butchers) the cutting, grinding, and proportioning of meat. Along the back wall or in the far corners, both for easy installation of refrigeration and back access to make for easy loading from the refrigerated trucks, is usually the dairy department.

That leaves the centre of the grocery store: the aisles and aisles of dry goods and manufactured packaged food.

Prior to World War II, most grocery stores were small, independently owned shops with limited floor space. The walls were often utilized the same ways they are now with butchers and refrigerated cases for dairy and eggs. In some places like the American South, the produce section was actually outside the store's doors in the form of carts and displays set up each day by the local farmers themselves, their wares determined by the season.

The central aisles carried staples like flours, oils, and seasonings, but were nothing like the great yawning mazes of aisle after aisle we see today. In the past two decades, grocery stores have exploded in sheer size. In suburban areas, grocery stores can take up anywhere from sixty to one hundred thousand square feet of retail space. This growth is nearly entirely dedicated to the variety of ultra-processed foods. A typical grocery store may even dedicate the entire length of a hundred-foot-long, ten-foot-high shelving space entirely to potato chips. There is no place where the predominance of grains and junk in our diets is more immediately apparent than your average grocery store.

In response to this trend, a common bit of advice has

cropped up for those looking to eat healthy: shop the edges.

While simple, this is strong advice! It allows you to focus on the foods that most closely resemble their form at harvest time, which is the best guideline to set yourself in order get the nutrition you need and avoid the temptation of addictive, disease-causing junk food. It's a great place to start and demonstrates that the changes you need to achieve your health goals don't have to be complicated. Stick to animal protein and seasonal produce for the vast majority of what ends up in your basket. If you're passing through a central aisle, limit yourself to olive oil and spices and get out.

You'll walk away having spent less money and time. And your body will thank you for it!

4

ENVIRONMENTAL SABOTAGE

Even before we are born, we are influenced and impacted by the environment around us. Our bodies and our minds are like sponges, taking in elements from the air we breathe, the surfaces we touch, and of course, the food we eat. In the modern world, our environments are like minefields, tainted with a growing number of toxic substances.

In 2010, the National Institute of Health and the National Cancer Institute reported that of the 80,000 manufactured chemical products in use and available in the market, only a few hundred of them have been tested for safety.[1] In the US and other developed countries, regulation in manufacturing has been largely reactionary rather than precautionary. And even the reactionary regulation is slow and requires too high a bar, as chemicals like "bisphenol A (BPA), is still found in many consumer products and remains unregulated in the United States, despite the growing link between BPA and several diseases, including various cancers."[2]

We are up to our necks in synthetic chemicals that are

too little understood to be so completely incorporated into our lives.

One of the most dangerous chemicals in widespread use is glyphosate, most commonly found in popular weed-killers like Roundup®.[3]

In 1961, the Stauffer Chemical Company patented glyphosate as a descaling and chelating agent. Initially, its primary use was as a descaling agent to clean out calcium and other mineral deposits in pipes and boilers of residential and commercial hot water systems. The strong metal-chelating properties of glyphosate allowed it to bind to calcium, magnesium, and heavy metals, making them water-soluble and easily removable.

What was initially designed to break down hard deposits off metal pipes—a harsh and industrial chemical —found its way over the next few decades into common use in agriculture and into one of the most basic staples of our food supply: grain.

In 1970, Monsanto scientist John Franz identified its herbicidal properties and patented it. Four years later, Monsanto introduced glyphosate to the market under the trade name Roundup. Over the next few decades, this herbicide became a standard in both commercial and private use. By the writing of a 2016 study for *Environmental Sciences Europe*, over 1.6 billion kilograms of glyphosate active ingredient has been applied in the United States alone since 1974.[4] As Monsanto increased the use of the harsh chemical in the late twentieth century, they also developed genetically modified corn and hybridized wheat strains to withstand and survive the effects of the herbicide, allowing mass farming operations to use the product more heavily and indiscriminately, increasing its presence in the soil. The claims that the substance does not end up in groundwater and run-off are dependent on how the substance adheres to soil, but this ignores how the product accumulates in the soil over time.

In the early 2000s, it was patented a third time (by Monsanto again) as an oral antibiotic. All these applications impact human health in a negative way.

Parallel to glyphosate's rise were studies of its effects on human, animal, and environmental health. The conclusion of a 2022 study summarized the effects of glyphosate exposure.:

Exposure to glyphosate during the early stages of life can severely affect normal cell development by deregulating some of the signalling pathways involved in this process....Glyphosate also seems to exert a significant toxic effect on neurotransmission, with the glutamatergic system being one of the most affected systems . . . it is unequivocal that exposure to glyphosate, alone or in commercial formulations, can produce important alterations in the structure and function of the nervous system of humans, rodents, fish, and invertebrate animals.[5]

Despite these devastating findings, the EPA's and Health Canada's position on glyphosate remains that it is safe to use "in accordance with its current label," but provides no way to enforce limiting its actual use to label-use.[6] Further, this ignores the high probability that its negative effects will increase over time through accumulation and long-time use. Although glyphosate has been banned in many places around the world, it is still heavily used in Canada and is the most commonly used herbicide among Canadian farmers. Crops like wheat, corn, and soy are the top uses, but chickpeas and oats are also heavily treated with it as well.

The Regulatory Challenges of Chemical Use

The Environmental Protection Agency (EPA) also recently relaxed restrictions of Chlormequat, an agricultural chemical used both as a general pesticide and to affect plant growth. When applied to oat and grain crops during their growth, it prevents the plants from bending over, making harvesting easier. Under the Trump administration, the EPA permitted Chlormequat residue on imported oats, leading to its presence in various food products. The EPA is now proposing to allow Chlormequat on domestic wheat and oats, potentially increasing its presence in our food.

Even without domestic use in the United States, Chlormequat is already highly present in both the food on the shelves and in our bodies. A study funded by the Environmental Working Group in 2023 detected the chemical in 92 percent of oat-based foods like Quaker Oats and Cheerios, and in the urine of 80 percent of people tested.[7] Because of our global food system, regulations by one nation are not enough to keep it out of the food that is mass-produced and distributed around the world. Chlormequat has already been in use in Canada, a major provider of wheat and oats to major food manufacturers throughout North America.

Exposure and consumption of Chlormequat have been linked to reproductive damage and fetal growth disruption in repeated animal studies.[8] While more research is needed to determine the level of effect in human exposure and consumption, it is highly probable that similar issues will appear. And yet, its use is currently being increased and expanded in our food supply and all around us, despite these findings.

Another pernicious class of chemicals embedded deeply in our environment is obesogens. Obesogens are a class of chemicals that can also be described as "endocrine-disrupting chemicals" or EDCs.[9] The class of chemical includes byproducts of plastics like Phthalates and Bisphenol A (BPA), chemicals used in non-stick coatings like Perfluorodecanoic Acid (PFOA), and agricultural chemicals like Organochlorines and Atrazine. They can be found in foods with high-fructose corn syrup and even in air pollution.

EDCs can mimic, block, or interfere with the body's hormones, leading to adverse health outcomes such as altered fertility, sex organ abnormalities, early puberty, nervous system dysfunction, immune issues, certain cancers, metabolic problems, obesity, cardiovascular conditions, and more.[10]

They are found in everyday household items like food containers, toys, cookware, personal care products, cleaning agents, and medical supplies. Because they're present in such a wide range of sources, they may contaminate food, water, or air, thereby further increasing their routes of exposure.

These chemicals are so pervasive in our environments that it can be very difficult to avoid them altogether. However, by limiting or eliminating your consumption of grains (the crops most often modified to withstand chemicals like glyphosate) and buying as much as possible from regenerative farms like those discussed in the previous chapter, or choosing organic you can significantly reduce your personal exposure to agricultural chemicals.

In your household, you can reduce plastics—especially plastic food storage containers—avoid cosmetics and cleaning products that contain these toxins, install and maintain air and water filters, and stick to non-toxic cook-ware like cast iron, stainless steel, and glass.

You can find more information on these chemicals through the Environmental Working Group (EWG).[11] The EWG is an American activist group that works to reduce harmful chemicals in our environment. They also provide manufacturers who avoid all the chemicals listed as chemicals of concern to human health or the environ-ment with the EWG certified label. The label appears on products that adhere to a much stricter code of require-ments than that required for approval by the Environ-mental Protection Act (EPA or the CEPA). It is a useful guidepost in stores when selecting products, especially skin care and cleaning supplies. With some time, patience, and research, you can significantly reduce the concentration of these chemicals in your home and your family's exposure to them.

For broader action, the EWG also accepts donations to aid in their campaigns to reduce the industrial use of harmful chemicals, both through private sector pressure on manufacturers and stricter government regulation. For those who want to help but cannot do so financially, they also frequently organize petitions and letter-writing campaigns to urge American institutions and global producers to actively curtail the proliferate use of these chemicals in our environment, especially in the produc-tion of our food.

The Effects of Environmental Poisons on Children

Children often suffer the worst side effects of toxic expo-sure. The concentration of exposure is higher, with greater exposures per kilogram of body weight compared to adults. Their physiological needs for food, water, and air are higher, so they take in more from their environments. Even from the protection of the womb, exposure to chemical pollutants can cause changes in organ system functioning, metabolic capabilities, and physical size of developing fetuses.

This is made ever more difficult because children also have the least amount of autonomy and choice when it comes to their environments.

Kids are heavily impacted by our modern food system. Because there is so much confusion around food and how far we've moved away from ancestral ways of eating, today's youth are now among the unhealthiest generation of kids to be born.

In a 2022 analysis of changing children's health, Jose Saavedra noted, "In 1990, child wasting was the #1 leading risk factor for mortality for all ages, and high body mass index (BMI) was #16; today, they are #11 and #5, respectively." While global childhood hunger is decreasing through efforts to provide food to developing nations and food security programs, the food most readily provided to these vulnerable populations is nutritionally deficient, which accounts for both this flip-flop in the causes of childhood mortality and the across-the-board decline in childhood health.

It's hard to imagine a generation of children with both more food and more undernourishment, but that is exactly the state that they are in. The effects are in their bodies, but also in their minds and culture. Children with poor nutrition do worse in school, simply because it's much harder to think clearly and maintain focus and awareness when you're malnourished.

Researchers have been measuring a steady rate of

decline in children's physical health since the turn of the century. Children are less able to run, with both speed and endurance showing steady declines. These aerobic movements are crucial in developing the lung capacity and musculature necessary in adulthood. Children who struggle with or get insufficient aerobic exercise as children are far more likely to struggle with cardiovascular health as adults.

Stress caused by poor physical health and struggles with academic performance can subsequently lead to higher rates of drug and alcohol use and even participation in crime. Lack of access to quality diet and exercise is the starting point for many lifelong mental, physical, and social issues.

There is also a rise in chronic, metabolic diseases in children, including the dangerous but difficult-to-detect NAFLD, or non-alcoholic fatty liver disease. According to the American Liver Foundation, the number of children affected by fatty liver disease is on the rise having more than doubled in the last twenty years. Today, approximately one in ten children is affected by NAFLD.[12]

NAFLD is a dangerous condition because while it can be invisible and symptomless for many years, scarring can develop over time and result in NASH, or non-alcoholic steatohepatitis. Dr. Charina Ramirez, a pediatric gastroenterologist at Children's Health, has been raising awareness of this issue for many years. In an article for Children's Health, Dr. Ramirez noted that "NASH is now the number one reason for liver transplantation in women, and in men, it's the second leading cause of transplantation behind alcoholic liver disease."[13] This rise is largely due to symptoms that begin undetected in childhood.

Lifestyle Changes to Counter Environmental Toxins

While there is no medical treatment or reversal for liver scarring and NASH, the liver is a regenerating organ, and the effects of NAFLD can be reversed if action is taken before scarring occurs.[14] Changes in diet and lifestyle are the most effective preventive steps for liver disease and associated metabolic disorders.

These changes can be difficult if not impossible for children to make on their own due to their lack of autonomy in food choices. Most school-provided lunches rely on packaged or heavily processed food and are deficient in protein. Children are also most susceptible to advertising and the social pressure to enjoy the most convenient foods that immediately satisfy cravings from sugar, processed grain, and other addictions.

While we cannot individually make radical changes in the global environment, we can make mindful choices about the immediate environment of our children and families. Children are absolutely the products of their environment, but we can mindfully improve that environment. By making the choices described above for ourselves, we can extend them to the household. By providing an example of a healthy lifestyle and a home where it is easier to achieve, we can ensure the best possible chance for our children to grow into strong and happy adults who will continue good habits their whole lives.

As a species, we move less than ever before.

Paradoxically, we also *rest* less than ever before.

Everything from developments in screen technology to the growth of car-centric urban environments has led to a lot of sitting in Western culture. This sedentary lifestyle is at odds with our evolutionary development.

In addition to a growing lack of exercise, many are moving away from a clear meal structure toward eating throughout the day. Originally suggested as a way to mitigate cravings while dieting and consume fewer calories overall, the true effects of eating small meals or snacks several times a day are quite the opposite. Cravings for foods with addictive properties don't decrease with frequency of use, but *increase,* leading to small snacks growing to larger "snacks." More empty calories throughout the day lead to less satisfaction and less room for nutrient-dense meals centred on animal protein. Additionally, this method of eating never provides our digestive tracts a break. Over time, this can weaken its ability to extract the most valuable nutrients from our foods.

Our ancestors spent most of their time outdoors where they were constantly exposed to sunlight, which helps set our circadian rhythm for better sleep and which stimulates natural production of vitamin D. Today, vitamin D deficiency is a major risk more and more people stay indoors for days at a time. Vitamin D deficiency is a common risk factor for cardiovascular disease.[15]

While we move less and stay inside more, modern lifestyles often do not correlate with more restorative rest, but rather longer (seated) working hours, recreation that is not restorative to our bodies or mental health, and disrupted and insufficient sleep.

In future chapters, we will explore the benefits of getting outdoors and finding our connection with nature as well as finding space for true, low-stimulation rest. But first, we'll look into the enormous benefits of movement and mindful exercise.

Our evolutionary ancestors moved frequently throughout their lives, both in bursts of intensity and in long efforts of stamina and endurance. Without this movement, our muscle density and structure suffer greatly. Of course, this deterioration of muscle makes us physically weaker, slower, less flexible, and more easily fatigued. But these obvious physical signs are not the only drawbacks to lower muscular development.

Dr. Gabrielle Lyon outlines the link between muscular health and metabolic health in her book *Forever Strong: A New, Science-Based Strategy for Aging Well.*[16] Dr. Lyon started her career with research that examined both nutritional science and geriatric studies. She also worked in an obesity clinic for two years and grew more and more frustrated as she could see the standard advice for weight management was failing to produce any real or lasting effects for her patients. Many such clinics are revolving doors of patients focused intently on losing weight, following all the guidelines they are given, and repeatedly failing. This doesn't help their physical health and damages their self-worth and mental health.

Dr. Lyon asked herself: "Why, with all our scientific insights, are we still chasing obesity?"

Through her research, Doctor Lyon realised that perhaps the problem was not that we are over-fat, but that we are under-muscled. By shifting our focus on building muscle rather than burning fat, we can build health not just in physical ability, but also in metabolic health and our immune systems. It is the key to metabolic health because healthy muscle mass not only changes your physical structure but also directs how your body uses both food and energy.

Through building muscle density, we increase the density of muscle mitochondria, the most important energy producing units within almost every cell of the body. In turn, this gives your body more energy to metabolize food and use the nutrients effectively.

When we strength train, we are also boosting our immune systems because muscle contraction releases peptides into our system. Peptides are short chains of amino acids. These molecules play various essential roles in the body, acting as signalling molecules and regulators of biological processes. They can stimulate cell growth in every system of the body, improving neural pathways, immune responses, and bone density.

Studies have shown that in as quickly as two weeks, introducing strength training into your lifestyle can improve blood sugar regulation, aid in digestion—which increases satiety after meals—and increase mobility. While it might be difficult to get started with a training program, especially starting from a very sedentary lifestyle, my clients find that the knowledge that they will soon start to feel better is a great motivation.

The long-term benefits of muscle training are even more essential to health and longevity. You can have stronger bones with decreased risk of osteoporosis.[17] You can lower your triglycerides which protects against heart disease.[18] You can strengthen your immune system, guarding against communicable diseases.[19] With more energy and better-regulated body chemistry, you will have better, more stable moods and feel happier, more capable, and more content more often.

With so many of us spending our working days

seated, hunched over a keyboard and our free time bent over a phone screen or lounged in front of a TV, eating empty foods continuously throughout the day, we could not be further divorced from the way our bodies are meant to consume, move, and feel.

To get back what we've lost, we need to be mindful about what we let into our bodies by keeping our diets as close to whole foods as possible. We should watch what we let into our homes and rub on our skin by making careful choices in what products we buy. And we must build a foundation of muscle by making time for the rigorous movement our bodies were made for.

5

IN THE MOOD

ONE OF THE foundational principles of physics is inertia.

Inertia is the resistance an object has to changes in its state of motion. An object at rest will remain at rest unless acted on by a significant force. Conversely, an object in motion will continue its direction and velocity until it is acted against in an opposite direction by a powerful force, often friction or gravity. The strength of the force needed to change an object's motion must be relative to the object's mass.

Our lifestyles are subject to a sort of inertia, too. We roll along with the momentum of habit, repeating the same things day after day. Just as an object resists changes to its motion, we often resist changes to our behaviour. Even if we recognize the need for improvement, it takes a significant push to break out of established habits and routines due to the inertia of familiarity. Even with a significant enough first push toward a healthier life, our old habits—like gravity—can easily pull us back.

Sustaining change requires motivation to keep going until our new speed becomes ingrained and inertia becomes a friend, keeping us going as though it were second nature.

To find the motivation needed to make permanent changes in our lifestyles, we need to connect and tune in to how our lifestyle, especially what we eat and how much we move, affects our daily mood. Mood is an invisible but powerful indicator of our overall health if we pay attention to its shifts and changes. When we tune into our mood, we can feel whether our lifestyle is getting in the way of our sense of well-being. And when we make the changes necessary to live a healthier lifestyle, one of the first changes is that invisible one—we *feel* better. Our mood changes more quickly and consistently than the measurable or physical changes to our bodies. Tuning into our mood, recognizing it, and celebrating it can provide that motivating force to keep going.

But first, we need to recognize how the status quo may be standing in the way of feeling better, often literally blocking the mental pathways to happiness.

Mood-Killing Foods

Our ability to feel good is deeply tied to what we eat.

The food we use to fuel our bodies provides the building blocks for our neurotransmitters, the chemicals in the brain that regulate mood. For example, the amino acids found in protein-rich foods are precursors to neurotransmitters like serotonin and dopamine, which are involved in mood regulation. Fluctuations in blood sugar levels, especially rapid spikes and crashes, can also influence mood. Consuming high-sugar foods or refined carbohydrates can lead to quick spikes in blood sugar followed by crashes, which may result in mood swings, irritability, and fatigue. Gut microbiota, the community of microorganisms living in the digestive tract, also plays a significant role in mood regulation. The gut microbiota communicates bidirectionally with the brain through the gut-brain axis, influencing neurotransmitter production, inflammation, and stress responses.

These complex systems in our bodies can all work in harmony to give us a persistent sense of well-being, or when out of balance and disjointed, make us feel anxious, helpless, and out of joint ourselves.

The grains-centric dietary advice that has been predominant since the 1970s does a terrible job of keeping these systems in a positive balance. I believe that building our food and our plates around grains first has sabotaged our diets and set us up for the need to have more and more processed grains and sugar - which is why it's so hard to say no to bread or that ice cream after dinner.

The problem with this food being foundational in our diets is that processed grains and sugar actually *wipe out* our nutrients. They deplete our body from essential B vitamins and vitamin C.[1]

In response to spikes in blood sugar, the body releases insulin to help regulate blood sugar. However, high levels of insulin can interfere with the absorption and utilization of B vitamins, particularly B1 (thiamine), B2 (riboflavin), B3 (niacin), B5 (pantothenic acid), and B6 (pyridoxine). These vitamins play a crucial role in the synthesis of neurotransmitters, which are essential in maintaining a positive chemical balance in the brain.

Similar to B vitamins, excessive sugar intake can also impact the body's utilization of vitamin C. When we consume sugar, it competes with vitamin C for uptake into cells. Elevated blood sugar levels can also increase inflammation, leading to greater utilization of vitamin C to neutralize free radicals and support immune function. High sugar intake burns up the nutrients in our systems, and it provides nothing in return but extra calories. In fact, processed grains act in the body exactly like sugar, so from this point on if I only refer to sugar - consider it the same for both processed grains and sugar.

The intake of sugar in the average diet has ballooned in recent decades, especially since the introduction of high-fructose corn syrup (HFCS).[2] Though HFCS has only been in use since 1980, we now make 17.5 billion pounds of it and consume sixty-six pounds per person per year. Dr. Mark Hyman outlines the devastating effects of sugar consumption not only on the body, but on the brain, in *The UltraMind Solution: Fix your broken Brain by Healing your Body First*.[3] In addition to robbing the body of nutrients, high sugar consumption has been tied to many mental disorders, including depression and anxiety. Over time, high sugar consumption can even cause crusting in your brain. As Hyman writes, sugar "reacts with proteins and forms little crusts or plagues called AGEs (advanced glycation end products). These crusty sugar-protein combos gum up your brain, leading to dementia."[4]

And that is just the physiological impact of sugar.

In *The Mood Cure*, Julia Ross names sugar as the number one "bad-mood food," also demonstrating how white-flour starches, even in foods that may be "savoury" to our palates, react with our body's chemistry in ways that mimic sugar.[5]

She also outlines the problems that wheat and other gluten-containing grains like rye, oats, and barley can cause. Gluten can cause inflammation of the digestive tract, which in turn can block the absorption of nutrients, leading to malnutrition, a root cause of many mental and physical ailments. Wheat grown in the United States is mostly a hybrid "developed specifically to increase gluten content so that baked goods will have more puff. But the hybridization has made it the most indigestible flour in the world."

While some people may be "immune" to the negative effects of gluten, the population of gluten-sensitive people may be much larger than we think, and only exacerbated by the introduction of hybrids that make its effects more acute and felt by a wider percentage of the population than in previous generations.

Eliminating the consumption of gluten has been successfully used as a treatment for people suffering from depression and manic depression in hospital settings. Those suffering from chronic exhaustion often turn to caffeine and stimulants for help, but eliminating gluten may have a longer-term positive effect on energy levels.

As we discussed in Chapter 1, gluten and sugar both cause a temporary spike in serotonin production, which does make us feel good for brief periods, just as the use of recreational drugs makes users feel good for a brief period after use. However, as with drug addiction, those spikes tend to decrease over time, straining the brain's ability to produce serotonin at a steady rate. Like any addiction, continuing to consume sugar and gluten because of the immediate sense of pleasure is trading long-term health for a short-term sensation.

Sugar isn't the only problematic food. Ross also identifies vegetable oils and other sources of trans fat as bad-mood foods.[6] Hydrogenated oils came into popular use in the 1960s as both a response to the cultural fear of saturated fats and the desire for a shelf-stable product. However, trans fats (fats transformed by the process of exposure to high heat and forced oxygen) cause far greater harm than any naturally occurring saturated fat in animal protein. They have cardiovascular impacts, and they directly affect the brain by producing an excess of Omega-6 fats. While Omega-6 is essential for our bodies to function, the concentrated levels contained in vegetable oils lead to a complete take-over of Omega-6 in the body, preventing the brain from using protective Omega-3 fats. This dysregulation can lead to mood disorders and depression.[7]

Over the past thirty years, there has been a steady increase in the prescribed use of antidepressants and other mood stabilizing medications, and this increase is only gaining momentum, especially among young people. In the past four years alone, antidepressant prescriptions for young adults have increased nearly 64 percent.[8] These medications can be enormously effective and useful for people struggling with mental health. However, most who are struggling to maintain a positive mood and general feelings of dissatisfaction may benefit more directly and permanently by eliminating these brain-damaging foods from their diets before seeking chemical aid.

The Dangers of Stillness

Just as our bodies are designed to consume natural foods, they are also built for natural movement. In short, we are built for motion.

Our early ancestors spent most of the day on the move

as hunters and gatherers, making camp in caves or where it was safe from predators. We avoided becoming prey by moving consistently throughout the day.

For millions of years, the subconscious mantra of our ancestors was to move or perish. And in reality, this is still true. Living a sedentary, largely still and unmoving lifestyle can still contribute directly to mortality—the process is just a bit slower than the jaws of a tiger. The previous chapter noted the importance of muscle and exercise on body chemistry and health, but movement is crucial to maintaining positive brain chemistry as well.

The reason is related to our ancestors' lifestyles. For early humans, moments of stress were acute reactions to danger. On a chemical level, our bodies do a relatively good job of responding to acute stress. In moments of fight or flight, cortisol increases in the brain, speeding up our metabolism so we have maximum access to the energy needed to escape or combat the clear and present danger. Once the danger has passed, cortisol levels return to normal. However, in our modern lifestyles, the stress is not as acute as it was for our ancestors. The stress of modern living is constant. There are few moments of immediate life-and-death danger, but continual societal pressures send our cortisol levels bounding in different directions constantly, never settling.

Worse still, this low level of stress is divorced from a need for physical movement. We aren't being chased by tigers, so the stress of modern living is rarely counteracted by physical movement. A 2018 study found that the majority of young adults in the United States sit for over nine hours per day.[9] Between the increase in desk work and screen-centric leisure time, the increased stillness of each generation increases the prevalence of chronic illness, both mental and physical.

A 2020 study collected responses from over twenty-eight thousand young people between the ages of eighteen and twenty and found a significant association between sedentary behaviour and anxiety, depression, and even suicidal behaviour.[10]

The dangers of still and seated lifestyles are significant for both physical and mental health, and the effects can be compounded over time, as deteriorating physical health can increase issues with mental health. In turn, poor mental health can create significant barriers to making the lifestyle changes needed to slow and reverse those negative health impacts. Stillness can create ruts around us, further limiting our movement and increasing the inertia effect, requiring greater and greater willpower to change direction.

Fortunately, there is some good news about movement—it can and will make you feel better, and it can show positive effects immediately.

The 2018 study for Preventive Medicine followed the daily movement and moods of 271 people. Participants wore a movement-recording armband that measured their sedentary time, their movement, and their sleep patterns first for a ten-day period and again one year later.[11] The participants also completed the profile of mood states and the perceived stress scale in order to measure mental well-being and changes in mood. The study confirmed what previous research had indicated: that more activity led to a greater sense of well-being and positive moods overall. By further examining the duration and frequency of movement with changes in mood on a daily basis, researchers further found that the effects of movement on mood were often immediate from one day to the next. More physical activity during the day also directly impacted the quality of sleep, both averaged over time and on a daily basis.

This is good news indeed, because to overcome the inertia effect and make lasting change, it is crucial to create a positive feedback loop that will continually give the motivation to keep going and fight the gravity of our old habits.

Get Moving, Stay Moving

One of the surest ways to sabotage efforts to improve both physical and mental health is to envision one, huge, monumental effort that will return the desired results and then allow us to return, victorious, to our typical way of life.

This is a setup for failure.

First, your monumental effort will almost certainly exhaust you well before you see the results you banked on. That disappointment will take the wind out of your sails and leave you worse off than you were before. And even if you *are* successful in achieving the result you wanted, going back to the lifestyle you had before will also send you back to the results you had before.

To improve both our mental and physical health, we need to get moving and *stay* moving.

This might sound easier said than done, but it is achievable with a solid plan. I know because I have seen it in my clients. To build up a sustainable exercise practice, start with manageable goals. Walking requires no special equipment other than good shoes, and a walking routine can be established at any level of physical ability. Our ancestors walked approximately six to sixteen kilometres per day, with walking making up the majority of their daily exercise. Start with one kilometre per day and be determined not to let excuses stop you.

Habits that aren't serving us are far from the only trap that must be avoided. Negative self-talk can generate many of the excuses that get in the way of our movement goals. We often tell ourselves that our new habits are too difficult, that we simply are not good at moving because we did not play sports as a young person, or that we have too little time to spare for it. Refuse to allow this negativity to get you started, and soon, with an elevated mood, you will find ways to gradually increase your activity and feel those increasingly beneficial effects.

We can also deliberately incorporate ways to replenish that motivational cup and build our momentum.

One way is to tap into our ancestral tribal instinct and join a community program to get additional exercise in a supportive group setting. In a 2009 study for the Mayo Clinic, researchers found that "exercise with one or more partners improves adherence and mood."[12] In other words, movement that involves community participation can increase the positive mood effects of activity, as social interaction can increase feelings of well-being and happiness.

Another way to increase positive feelings around exercise is to create and enjoy a variety of activities since this approach both challenges us to learn new styles of training and allows us to experiment and find the forms of movement we enjoy. For instance, incorporating resistance training into our movement routines is an easy step up that can decrease boredom and increase our feelings of accomplishment. There are many free videos online with twenty- or thirty-minute routines, either using weights and resistance or body weight alone. Laying the foundation for building muscle will increase your health in so many ways, from a stronger immune system to better sleep and improved mental health. When you start to feel better, you can draw on that feeling to keep going.

Mood-Boosting Through Food

The effects of activity on mood can also be compounded through diet to both accelerate results and increase the feelings of positivity around lifestyle changes. Just as certain foods block the mental pathways necessary to maintain good moods, there are foods that can improve our dispositions as well as our overall health. Like exercise, tuning into elevated moods and being sensitive to how food can alter your mental state can help provide the support needed to maintain a consistent and healthy diet.

Julia Ross identifies protein as the number one good-mood food. Without sufficient protein, it is literally impossible to feel "optimistic, enthusiastic, calm, or comforted."[13] The neurotransmitters that send out all these positive feelings can be made only by using amino acids. The more protein, the more our brains can feel well. Ross recommends concentrated sources of protein such as fish (which also contain brain-supporting Omega-3s), poultry, eggs, and red meat. These sources also contain the second good-mood food: good fats. Though concerns about fats are pervasive, the truth is that low-fat diets have not reduced heart disease in the general population. Fat also serves the crucial function of helping us feel *satisfied* from food, elevating our moods and ensuring what we eat is fulfilling both our nutritional and emotional need for sustenance.

Besides protein and fats, Ross also explains that many vegetables are good-mood foods. Our brains and bodies can benefit from *some* carbohydrates to function, and vegetables are a great form of carbohydrates that do not cause blood sugar spikes that throw off hormone and insulin balances throughout the body.

Your ability to feel *happy* lives in your brain and your gut. The key to enjoying more happiness, every single day, is to take away the barriers that interfere with your brain's function while supporting the elements it needs to run efficiently. A diet centred around animal-based protein, good fats, and vegetables that avoid processed sugars, vegetable oils, and processed grains will not only increase your health and longevity. It will also increase your daily happiness.

The first positive result of change is likely to be your mood. Through the combined efforts of increased movement and good food, your capacity for satisfaction and contentment can grow starting the very first day you make changes. I know because I have seen this in my clients, and I have seen it in myself. To keep the gravity of bad habits from pulling you back to the cycle of immediate gratification and addiction, it is essential to be sensitive to those first positive changes in mood. The first change is invisible, but it is palpable. Logging your mood and reflecting on how much *better* you can feel can give you the necessary force to build momentum toward your goals. Eventually, the newly adopted lifestyle will no longer be new, making it effortless to maintain.

With consistent effort, your inertia will shift forever increasing your capacity for happiness and satisfaction.

6

RECONNECT WITH OUR ANCESTORS

In our culture, misinformation can be subject to its own form of inertia. Bad advice, repeated often, becomes cemented in the collective understanding making it very difficult to dislodge.

We all understand that our bodies are complicated organisms, with myriad factors playing out at any given time between our different organ and cellular systems. Thankfully, these complex systems are all automatic—we don't have to tell our pancreas to manufacture hormones, our immune system to fight invading cells, or the mitochondria of our cells to produce energy any more than we must tell our hearts to beat. We couldn't micro-manage these systems even if we tried, but their efficiency is greatly affected by what we eat and how much we move.

We all know and understand this. And yet, we also know that we can't all be nutrition experts, spending our days figuring out exactly what to eat to serve each element of this incredibly complex system we call a body. Even if we could, doing so would soon create an unhealthy relationship with food. To sustain a healthy lifestyle over the long term requires simple guidelines that we can reasonably remember and follow, while still enjoying what we eat.

The best guideline for us to follow is to simply reconnect with the way our ancestors ate and moved, the way we *evolved* all those complex systems in the first place. As we have explored in previous chapters, our ancestors moved frequently throughout each day and got the majority of their calories from animal proteins with nutritional support from plant matter. They never ate refined carbs or sugars. Making our own lifestyles as close to our ancestors' as possible—and we can get closer than you might think—is the best way to ensure all our internal systems perform their intricate ballet as intended.

We can all support our health by providing what our bodies evolved to need.

So, if things are that simple, why do so few people adopt the ancestral lifestyle approach? Why is diet advice so convoluted and contradictory?

In some ways, it all comes back to inertia. The need for simple guidelines for diet and health has driven some scientists to the wrong conclusions, which translates quickly to bad advice. The more the advice is repeated, the deeper it burrows into our cultural understanding.

To make matters a hundred times worse, dietary advice is deeply tied to massive industries, and bad faith actors have direct influence on what "scientific" conclusions get translated into practical advice. In this chapter, we will look at the two "common-sense" pieces of diet advice that are rooted in terrible science. The sooner we can pry these rotten ideas out of the collective consciousness once and for all, the better for everyone.

The Saturated Fat Myth

Fat must make us *fat*. On the surface, it seems logical, even obvious. You are what you eat, ergo eating fat will make you fat.

Except this reasoning is not logical at all. The study of logic might call this an equivocation fallacy, a type of argument that *sounds* solid even though it is not. An equivocation fallacy occurs when a key term or phrase in an argument is used with different meanings in different parts of the argument, leading to a misleading or unsound conclusion. This fallacy exploits the ambiguity of language to make an argument appear more compelling than it actually is. For example, someone may say "a feather is light" and "what is light cannot be dark," ergo "a feather cannot be dark." When put like this, the fallacy is obvious. Two very different ideas, described by coincidence by the same word, cannot be connected to lead to a logical conclusion.

The exact same fallacy occurs when we conclude that eating fat makes us fat.

In her book *The Big Fat Surprise,* Nina Teicholz describes how pervasive and widespread this fallacy has become.

Has there ever been a more unfortunate homonym? One word means two very different things: the fat we eat and the fat on our bodies. It's so hard for our brains to fully grasp . . . fat in all forms has simply come to be commonly understood as something to be avoided. A large number of experiments have since confirmed that restricting fat does nothing to slim people down (quite the reverse, actually), yet even so, the idea that there could be such a thing as a "slimming fat" will probably always seem to us like an oxymoron.[1]

But this seemingly obvious completely false link could not have been so widely spread if it were only word play. It became so prominent because it was aggressively driven by industries and governmental agencies largely influenced by a single man—Ancel Keys.

Ancel Keys, though his degrees were primarily in animal biology, first became instrumental in questions of diet and nutrition during World War II. Keys spent much of the decade prior studying nutrition and energy, leading to the transformation of quantitative biology, particularly at high altitudes. After a relatively brief stint at the University of Minnesota, the US War Department recruited Keys to create easy-to-carry rations for parachute troops.[2]

One result was an incredibly calorie-dense food that was easy to carry, even when a person was jumping out of a plane. This was called the K-ration.

A second result was that Keys gained clout with the US government and the agencies that were being formed to study the relationship between diet and disease, particularly heart disease. Heart disease was growing into a primary concern as heart attacks were on the rise, though it was still a poorly understood phenomenon. By the mid-50s, Keys had developed the hypothesis that saturated fats were the primary cause of high cholesterol and associated heart disease. In a small study of psychiatric patients, Keys seemed to find evidence to support his theory. The study found that "serum cholesterol would go up after the men ate saturated fat and down after the vegetable oils."[3] Keys took this slim evidence and ran with it. He was so confident in his findings that he even proposed a mathematical formula for reducing cholesterol through diet and made sweeping recommendations to reduce saturated fats in diets across the board.

The fear of heart attacks intensified when US President Eisenhower suffered the first of a series of heart attacks. The President's doctor was a believer in Keys' work and cited him heavily when reporting both on the President's recovery and in response to questions about preventing heart disease. For the following decades, Keys would continue to maintain his hypothesis and dismiss or malign any evidence that called it into question, even within his own data. He championed the results found from the "Seven-Countries Study." Keys and his wife travelled and collected data from the USA, Finland, the Netherlands, Italy, Greece, Yugoslavia, and Japan. These cherry-picked countries did indeed show a correlation between saturated fats in diets and heart disease. While Keys would give the obligatory "correlation does not prove causation" caveat in his studies, he only doubled down on his advice to reduce saturated fats. His advice became the common standard pushed by government-supported agencies like the American Medical Association and American Heart Association. Industries responded with the developments of reduced-fat milk and oil-based alternatives like margarine. But further investigation shows that this conclusion is based on bad science, and it always has been.

Teicholz describes an early study by Doctors Yerushalmy and Hilleboe, which took in data from a broader and more diverse set of twenty-two countries. When considering all these countries, the clear line of correlation disappears into a scatter plot of points. In 1957, Yerushalmy further posited a number of other causes that could account for the same correlation including car pollution, cigarettes, and sugar consumption.

Keys dismissed this criticism out of hand and over the next several decades, continued to gather only data that would support his theory and dispute any other interpretation. In 1999, when it was demonstrated that sugar had an even more suggestive correlation in Keys's own original study, the scientist was outspoken against it and repeatedly dismissed concerns over sugar.

It is hard to understand why supposedly science-minded people like Keys could become so set on a single explanation that they would continuously dismiss all other concerns. Especially when there may be real consequences to over-stating the findings, considering that millions of people are still to this day adjusting how they eat according to his bombastic advice.

But the sugar industry had a vested interest in subduing any evidence that may link their product with bad health and shortened life span. In 2016, doctors concerned that funding from food industries was having an undue effect conducted a historical analysis of documents between sugar industrialists and scientific researchers and published their findings in *JAMA Internal Medicine*. The Sugar Research Foundation (SRF) was created by the sugar industry and for decades the SRF has funded study after study and review after review to discredit any negative findings about sugar, while ignoring any problems in studies that implicate fat as a cause of diet-related disease.[4]

These publications, collectively, have cemented the relationship between consumed fat and ill health in the collective understanding, despite that relationship being based on weak and misleading evidence. There has been enormous damage done by these practices, as diet-related disease is only on the rise as millions still restrict valuable foods like fats and substitute them with altered or synthetic low or no-fat alternatives. In his book *Fat for Fuel,* Dr. Joseph Mercola outlines how harmful these dietary guidelines may have been over the last seventy years: "No one knows for sure just how many premature deaths have resulted from this low-fat diet recommendation, but my guess is that this number is easily in the hundreds of millions."

In the same decades since these guidelines were adopted, diabetes, cancer, and heart disease have all been on the rise. Between 1978 and 2013, rates of diabetes in the US quadrupled from 5.19 million to 22.3 million. Cancer diagnoses have also risen significantly. While death rates from heart disease have declined because of advances in medical treatment and response, heart disease instances are also rising, with over a third of the population living with cardiovascular disease since 2010.[5]

While the established health advice demonized fat loudly and repeatedly, government-subsidized corn and sugar industries have intertwined intense concentrations of sugar in hundreds of the so-called "healthy" foods sold.

The Fibre Man

The glorification of dietary fibre has a similar origin, with one man pushing an over-reaching hypothesis well beyond its usefulness or appropriate scope. Researchers for Cambridge University investigated the history of fibre research and how it is centred primarily on a surgeon who would become known as the "fibre man": Dr. Denis

Burkitt. Burkitt observed significant differences in disease prevalence between Western populations and those in rural Africa. He noticed that diseases such as colorectal cancer, appendicitis, diverticular disease, and coronary heart disease were rare among African populations, who consumed a high-fibre diet predominantly consisting of unprocessed plant foods.

Burkitt hypothesized that the low incidence of these diseases in African populations was linked to their diet, which was rich in dietary fibre. This led to the formulation of the dietary fibre hypothesis, suggesting that a high intake of fibre helps to maintain bowel health, prevent constipation, and reduce the risk of developing chronic diseases, including congenital heart disease (CHD), diabetes, appendicitis, various vascular disorders, and even cancer.[6]

Burkitt's work influenced dietary guidelines for decades, but more recent and robust research calls into question the value of fibre—a substance we can scarcely call food since our body does not absorb it—in preventing disease. In a 2007 study, Kok-Yang Tan and Francis Seow-Choen reexamined Burkitt's studies and the research since and found that confounding factors weakened the suggested link between high-fibre diets and reduced disease risk. In further study, they concluded that dietary fibre did not protect against colorectal polyps, cancer, or even chronic constipation. In short, fibre did little to live up to Burkitt's initial claims.[7]

While dietary fibre is not significantly harmful in ways vegetable oils, processed grains, and sugars are, we should be skeptical about its necessity in our diets considering how much we are expected to consume today as compared to what some of our ancestors would have had access to. Not all our ancestors were eating fifty to a hundred grams of fibre per day, especially when you consider that plant foods were mostly eaten seasonally. There is more and more observational research being conducted that for some people, eliminating plant food for a short time can be healing under certain health conditions—and I have seen this personally in my practice too.

Plant-based fibre may have some palliative benefits to our digestive tract. But while many assume that dietary fibre is the single most important protection against digestive disease, modern scientific findings do not support this claim.

Saturated Fats are not Just Good for Us—They're Necessary

Far from being the heart-clogging killer they are maligned to be, saturated fats actually have enormous health benefits. Mercola explains in *Fat for Fuel* that fats are essential for our mitochondria to produce energy efficiently. They can also, perhaps somewhat counterintuitively, *improve* your cholesterol. The confusion around cholesterol stems from the fact that there are two kinds of lipoproteins we focus on when we run lipid blood tests and look at our cholesterol: high-density and low-density (HDL and LDL). HDL is now commonly considered "good" cholesterol and LDL is considered "bad," but it is even further complicated by the fact that LDL is also in multiple different forms—smaller, dense LDL particles and larger "fluffy" particles. The small, dense particles are the ones that contribute to higher risk of heart disease. Eating saturated fat can change the dangerous LDL into the "fluffy" kind, while eating refined sugar and grains increases the number of dangerous LDL particles.

In his book, Mercola also lists the additional health benefits to consuming saturated fats:

- They provide the building blocks for cell membranes, hormones
- They help to absorb minerals like calcium
- They carry our fat-soluble vitamins (A, D, E, K) around the body
- They are converters and convert nutrients like carotene into vitamin A
- They help lower very small dense lipoprotein (the problematic fat in our bodies) (through the fatty acids called palmitic and stearic acid)
- They act as antiviral agents (through the fatty acid called caprylic acid)
- They provide the optimal fuel for your brain when fats are converted to ketones
- They help you to feel full and satiated which means you're less likely to overeat and snack on processed food
- They help to modulate our genetics through epigenetics, which can aid in cancer prevention (through the fatty acid called butyric acid)
- They help to increase the beneficial large and fluffy LDL cholesterol which is not associated with the risk of heart disease
- Boosts HDL cholesterol which is touted as the beneficial cholesterol

- Saturated fats help to fuel our mitochondria (the powerhouse of our cells) and produce far fewer free radicals which damage the endothelial cells of our arteries.

With this long list of benefits, could we be causing more harm than good by following dietary guidelines of building our plates on plant foods and actively avoiding animal foods that contain beneficial saturated fat?

Saturated fats can also increase our pleasure and satisfaction from food, helping us maintain a healthy diet over the long term.

This should not be surprising. Our ancestors would have eaten a good deal of saturated fat. But this, too, is a misconception in our culture.

Saturated fats got their bad name unfairly and without rigorous support by careful science, but the nutritional myth persists and muddies the waters of other dietary research.

Revisiting Ancestral Diets

There has been growing interest over the last twenty years in eating according to ancestral practices, largely based on studies that show modern populations that eat according to these old traditions are far healthier and more robust compared to their counterparts, even close genetic relatives, who eat modern diets.

In the 1930s, Dr. Weston Price was a dentist who studied native populations and their diets and published his findings in "Nutrition and Physical Degeneration" in 1939. He was first drawn to study these populations through his dentistry practice, as Price observed that Indigenous peoples who followed traditional diets had excellent dental health, characterized by straight teeth, minimal cavities, and well-developed dental arches. In contrast, individuals who adopted modernized diets, high in refined sugars and processed foods, exhibited a higher prevalence of dental issues such as cavities, dental crowding, and tooth decay. Expanding his view, Price also found that they showed lower rates of chronic diseases such as heart disease, cancer, and arthritis compared to those consuming modernized diets. These populations often displayed higher levels of vitality, fertility, and resistance to infectious diseases. Price posited that this difference could be attributed to the main thing that made these populations' lifestyles different: their diets.[8]

His findings inspired many to try to adopt an ancestral lifestyle. However, these attempts were largely corrupted by misinformation. Through the sixties and seventies, proponents of the low-fat diet claimed that wild game was naturally low in saturated fats in comparison to raised livestock. While this might be partially true, researchers Fallon and Enig demonstrate the many issues with this analysis. For one thing, wild animals are high in saturated fats. Fallon and Enig compared the fat composition of many North American species of animals and found only a few smaller species, like squirrels, actually exemplify a lower level of saturated fat than cattle. More common game animals like deer have much higher rates of saturated fats.

They further looked at the real practices of these native peoples to illustrate saturated fats were not only readily consumed but prized. As has long been documented in the records of early explorers, many North American native populations sought out older animals to slaughter. This was not an accident—these populations preferred older animals because, through the aging process, these animals develop a substantial strip of fat that runs along their backs. Between this strip and the space around the internal organs, every thousand pounds of animal could yield up to eighty pounds of highly saturated fat. For many tribes, this resulted in diets that were made up of 80 percent fat by calories.[9]

There is increasing evidence that those who consume a diet most similar to our ancestral diets, in conjunction with an active lifestyle, have healthier outcomes than those who eat a modern diet, especially one high in vegetable oils, starches, and sugars. However, trying to combine this evidence with the faulty and corrupted evidence aggressively pushed by scientists like Ancel Keys creates contradictions and confusion. What was once proposed as a nutritional panacea now muddies the waters of what we actually know, leaving many of us with anything but a simple path to follow.

Letting go of nutritional myths and overcoming our fears of saturated fat can help us find that simple guideline that will truly work because it is based on thousands of years of wisdom passed down through the generations.

When it comes to your health, there is a lot of confusion, because of misinformation, about what the right choice is in terms of the "right" diet. I'm a proponent of individual choices based on your unique symptoms, not general dietary advice. There is no one-size-fits-all approach. For some people, high animal protein and less plant-based food is healing. For others, less animal food and more plant foods may be the best option. My advice: decide based on how you feel and what your blood work shows. And while you're at it, find a healthcare practitioner who understands the nuance of current nutrition research.

7

YOU ARE WHAT YOU EAT

For many years, I struggled with intense anxiety without understanding why.

I would have panic attacks, often in the car heading from one errand to the next. It would start as a feeling of unease that I could not quite place. The space in the car around me would seem to grow too close. I would start to feel trapped or threatened. My chest would tighten, and I struggled to get enough air. My heart pounded hard and fast. Suddenly, my body was on high alert, and I had no idea why. There was never any perceivable immediate threat to me, and yet my body was pumping hard in fight-or-flight. I could find no physical reason, either. My heart was healthy, I exercised regularly, and I could think of no objective reason why I was experiencing these horrible spells.

One day, I had this intuitive feeling that the problem could be mental, so I sought out therapy for my anxiety. From my very first appointment, therapy changed the way I looked at my life and my choices.

My therapist asked me to define and reflect on my

values. She asked me to consider the ways my life was aligned with my values and the ways it was not.

The prompt was desperately needed at that time in my life and when I considered this and re-aligned some of my values - it created an immediate feeling of calm in my chest.

I have always tried to live thoughtfully, but I had never quite thought about values like this. Through therapy, I realised that some of my feelings of panic and loss of control were rooted in small disconnects between my personal values and my daily choices. We are affected so much by our surroundings and society. When social expectations grate against the values and priorities we hold most dear, of course it creates stress.

Reflecting on this question took some time, and I still consider it every day. As I make big decisions or build the habits that shape my life, I let my core values guide me and help me resist choices that might be easy and frictionless, but that do not align with what I care about most.

Through this practice, my values have allowed me to develop my own personal code of conduct for trying to build a better micro-world for me and my family—based on what I believe are the most important ways of living—to achieve my goals of health, contentment, and personal success.

The foundation of my value system is to ensure I am truly being nourished. Being nourished is the foundation that allows me to dream big and have the energy to follow through.

My value system also acknowledges that I am intricately interconnected with nature and the greater world, and that the choices I make not only affect my health but the health of my environment. Being aligned with the natural world is a basic fundamental value of mine where I look to nature for answers in what is best for humanity as well as our ecosystem. This also requires that I make intentional choices about where I get my food. Focusing on small, local farms allows me to be personally nourished, while also considering all the impacts of farming on the soil, the environment, and the micro-economy.

I am not alone in having these values, but there are so many large systems in place that make it difficult for us to make these fundamental changes. Still, as challenging as they may be, those changes are *not* impossible.

One of the biggest obstacles my clients face when beginning to eat true to their values is expense. It is true that some foods come with a higher price tag when they are developed with good practices, but as we discussed in Chapter 3, there are many offsets that help make these practices affordable. Buying far too much cheap, convenient food not only misaligns with my values (and most of the values we all share!), but it wastes money that we could be deliberately using to better nourish ourselves.

Reading the ingredient list is really the only true method of knowing what is in manufactured food, and even then, we may not recognize the harms of substances that appear in nearly all manufactured foods, like vegetable oils.

More than following what producers put on packaging, the best rule of thumb is to focus most on foods that do not even have an ingredient list because they are whole, fresh, and unprocessed.

It is worth mentioning that a higher price tag does not necessarily translate to quality, nourishing, values-driven foods. Avoiding the inflated costs of so-called "healthy" packaged food can leave room in our budgets for true quality that aligns both with our dollar and moral value.

Health-Washing

As much as I prioritize getting my produce and meat mostly direct from local farms, there is of course no way to totally avoid the grocery store. There are some stores in my area that carry locally farmed meat and wonderful eggs and dairy. There are also basic essentials like olive oil and spices which are the simple keys necessary to make whole foods come together as a delicious meal.

But other than that, I stick to the outer walls of grocery stores, because even in "natural" health-food stores, the central aisles are full of packaged goods that are laden with unhealthy ingredients. These "healthy" versions of packaged food are bedazzled in buzzwords with eye-catching fonts: Non-GMO, Organic, All-Natural, Vegan, No Added Sugars, Low-Fat, Gluten-Free, Whole Grain, Fortified, Low-Calorie, Guilt-Free.

Meanwhile, these packages contain the same highly processed, manufactured "foods" that provide more mouthfeel than they do nutrition. Even "healthy" manu-factured brands have stockholders to please, so they strive for that bliss point that keeps people coming back, just as the non-health-oriented brands do. Their buzzword labels function primarily as workarounds that allow them to access the marketing clout provided by earning shelf space in the health-food stores.

This marketing strategy is called "health-washing," or the practice of using misleading or exaggerated claims about the health benefits of products to attract health-conscious consumers.[1]

Health-washing is all about the bait and switch. Some health-associated terms have no regulations around their use and can generally be considered meaningless. The worst of these culprits is the term "all-natural" which may preclude artificial food colouring, but otherwise has little to no real meaning on a label.[2]

Other ways manufacturers bait and switch is to apply labels that indicate health goals while hiding harmful additives or a simple lack of real nutrition. This practice may have had its origin during the scare over saturated fats. Manufacturers love applying the "low-fat" label to reduced-fat dairy products, snacks, and cheeses while loading these products with sugar and other additives to compensate for the lack of flavour. Similarly, the "sugar-free" label is a near guarantee of the addition of artificial sweeteners and chemicals to mimic the sensation of sweetness, a result that gives the same addictive effect as sugar. The fact that these foods usually taste a bit flat or off seems to further convince buyers that the food must be healthier.

Other labels like "whole grain" may be fully well-intended but allow manufacturers a lot of room for fudging. According to the Food and Drug Administration (FDA), whole grains must contain the entire grain seed or kernel, which includes the bran, germ, and endosperm. While it is true that these forms of grain have a greater concentration of vitamins and nutrients than their processed cousins, it does not necessarily mean that our bodies can absorb these nutrients effectively. Whole grain foods also contain more fibre. Many people believe this is a clear signal of healthy foods, but our needs for fibre have been greatly exaggerated and more likely varies widely based on individual need, since some people react negatively with too much fibre. Finally, to earn the label "whole grain" only 51 percent of the ingredients must be whole grain by weight, meaning up to 49 percent can be the processed or "white" forms of the grains. Manufacturers can tweak their processes just enough to earn the label, while still providing products that are very nearly half the highly processed starches that people seeking out whole grain foods are trying to avoid.

Other terms like "no added sugars" are linguistic workarounds meant to downplay naturally occurring or even *concentrated* sugars in fruit-based products.

Take food that may "qualify" for all these labels: Vegan, non-GMO, Organic, All-Natural, No Added Sugars, Artisan, Small-Batch, and Gluten-Free.

There are a lot of characters on that package aimed at convincing you that what is inside is good, nutritious, and safe. And yet, it may in fact be potato chips, deep fried in nut oils, and heavily salted. They provide some starchy calories, but no real nutrients. The hot oil treatment can be damaging to your arterial walls, and the combination of salt, crunch, starch, and fat make the chips sensationally satisfying and addictive. They keep you coming back for more and more, all while providing little other than calories that are quickly spent, leaving you craving more and more. Spending the extra money on these products because of these labels may avoid some of the nastier ingredients in traditional packaged foods, but this is no substitute for the nutritional value of real, whole foods.

These branding tactics have been in place for many years, both on food labels and in food advertising, because they are highly effective. One study examined how powerful simple food labelling can be on purchasing choices. The study focused on foods that were advertised as being "vitamin-fortified."[3]

Vitamin fortification, on the surface, sounds like a positive step a manufacturer can make, but in truth, it is at best an empty gesture and at worst a dangerous practice. Foods can only be "fortified" with vitamins if they are highly processed, and often these forms of the vitamins are synthetic or derived from non-ideal sources. The added vitamins usually are not as bioavailable (easily absorbed and used by the body) as those naturally occurring in foods. Additionally, the overall balance of nutrients is never as ideal as it would be in whole foods that naturally contain a variety of vitamins and minerals. Some foods may be "fortified" beyond what is necessary to consume at any given time, and this can lead to dangerous toxicity, especially if consumers ingest these synthetic concentrations of vitamins from multiple sources.

Because of this, the US FDA discourages the practice, especially in snack foods where "fortification" may be used as a health incentive on foods that otherwise have no health value at all, like cookies, chips, and carbonated beverages. Still, the practice remains widespread, and worse, incredibly effective with consumers.

A study published by the Journal of the Academy of Nutrition and Dietetics sought to assess the effect of this label on consumer decisions.[4] The study's participants were presented with a choice of snack foods. The foods had been secretly rated on a scale of "healthy" to "unhealthy," but the labels appeared to the consumers as they would in stores. Among the spread of snack foods, one food was labelled "fortified" with vitamins. However, in most sets of choices, the actual "healthiest" option was not the fortified option, as the fortified option had higher sugars and trans fats than the other foods.

The study found that not only were consumers most likely to choose the "vitamin-fortified" product over the others; if such a product were available, they were less likely to even *look* at the ingredients list or nutrition label, making their selection automatically.[5] They were also more likely to self-assess their purchase as the healthiest, even though there were healthier options available.[6] In other words, manufacturers do not have to do much to make their products *seem* like the healthier choice.

Additional studies have examined the effects of advertising, especially social media advertising which is currently the most influential form. The health-washing of products can range from misleading labelling to ads that feature subtle health cues. A snack commercial for a product full of additives and processed grains can feature a series of athletes performing amazing feats of agility and speed and then biting into the product with relish. A sugary drink may be handed to a runner on a marathon accompanied by subtle music changes, indicating through the power of suggestion that the drink is responsible for getting the athlete across the finish line. Some studies indicate that this suggestive health-washing imagery is included in over half of ads for ultra-processed foods.[7]

The good news is that studies also indicate that even a *little* information can go a long way in negating the effects of health-washing. A study published in Health Promotion International sought to measure the effects of receiving prior health information on the perception of products whose ads contained health-washing language or imagery. They included hundreds of adult individuals with a range of formal education who were all active on social media. The study found that those who were exposed to health information far more readily saw through brand manipulation and even held a negative association with health-washed products.[8]

To get through the day, consumers need simple, easy-to-follow guidelines to make the best choices for their health. Manufacturers take full advantage of this, selling the health label over actual, quality products. However, as we can see, knowing what to look for can easily arm us against such low-level manipulation and allow us to make better choices for our health.

The only way to really put an end to these misleading practices is to build communities that refuse to be fooled by them. That starts with your own dollars and how you spend them.

Value-Driven Economics

I found that the more I live in alignment with my values, the more at peace I feel, and this is especially true for things that I consume. When you take something into your body, it becomes a part of you. Feeling the best I possibly can about what I eat—both in terms of how it makes me feel and its effect on my environment—is essential for me to feel aligned with what I care about most. While the impact of my personal choices may be limited, I can make sure that the impact is a positive one. The small farms I order from and the sustainability-driven producers I patronize are empowered to keep going because of my choice. The more of us who make those deliberate choices over the convenient ones, the greater the positive impact. The greater the positive impact, the more convenient, available, and affordable those options may become. And as those choices become more widely available, more and more people can and will choose better for themselves and their communities, raising the status quo of our communities to a higher, healthier, and more sustainable level.

Collectively, our purchasing power can change the direction of our market economy to a more socially responsible economy, making food choices fair for everyone, and forcing companies to develop their own operating values based on reducing overfishing in our oceans and ending the confined animal feeding operations. Most importantly, we may be able to reverse the trend of single crops destroying soil health and emitting too much CO_2.

In his book, *Value(s): Building a Better World for All*, Mark Carney, the UN Special Envoy on Climate Action and Finance, shines a spotlight on many of the foundation-deep cracks in our society, from economic inequality (and the food insecurity that inevitably follows) to the looming crisis of climate change.[9] He centres his argument on another equivocation fallacy—this time not on "fat" but on "value." In our market-driven culture, "value" more often indicates the market price of something as opposed to the word's moral meaning. Carney emphasizes that markets need to be reminded that what society actually wants—health, fairness, and the preservation of natural beauty, diversity, and resources of our planet—cannot be reduced to a number. He does not sugarcoat the massive issues this imbalance has created and focuses on three global crises that illustrate the problem—the financial and credit crises, the flawed COVID-19 response, and climate change. Carney asks,

"How do we learn to be moral again? Markets (even food markets) were made to serve us; we were not made to serve markets. Economics needs ethics. Markets do not survive by market forces alone. They depend on respect for the people affected by our decisions. Lose that and we lose not just money and jobs but something more significant still; freedom, trust and decency, the things that have value, not a price."[10]

As an expert with decades of experience in global finance, Carney understands the gravity of these problems but is also highly optimistic that a truly values-based economy can be brought about through collective action and social pressure. It may not feel possible as we roam through the grocery store, with its aisles of cheap, non-nutritious foods and cases of CAFO-bred meat. The food system status quo is a behemoth, after all, and most of us are just trying to get through our days unscathed.

However, our values are also our deepest and truest sources of motivation. As we have discussed in previous chapters, inertia is powerful and change is hard. Our values are the core of who we are and who we want to be, and connecting to them as we make daily choices—not just the big decisions, but the everyday decisions about what we put in our bodies and homes—can help us make those hard changes easier and more sustainable. We may at first be only shaping our own bodies and immediate environments, but that small impact can and will ripple out into something much more powerful.

8

THE CASE FOR BOREDOM

The temperature in your area will be seven degrees warmer tomorrow.

An item in your cart has changed price. Hurry and buy now so you don't miss out on this deal.

Congratulations! You have reached your step goal.

Your Instagram post has thirteen new interactions, open app for more details.

The average adult receives around forty-six notifications on their phone a day,[1] usually confined to their waking hours as determined by phone usage.

Nearly four dings or buzzes per waking hour, calling for our attention and often asking for our immediate engagement or response.

This single aspect of our modern culture alone creates a huge amount of noise in our environments and our minds. As a culture and as a species, this constant flow of stimuli is very new to us. Many of us even experienced this stimulation as a new occurrence within the span of our lifetimes. This is not good for our sense of well-being, our creative abilities, or our mental health.

For teenagers, the issue is even worse. Teens average more than two hundred notifications per day, notifications that come in day and night, given that teens are more likely to engage with their phones regardless of the hour.[2]

The buzzing of a phone impacts our minds very differently than the buzzing of a bee as it bobs like a fat helicopter from flower to flower. The issue is not the sound itself, of course, but the response that sound triggers in our brains.

Cultural Obsession with Productivity

Increasingly over the last century, our culture has pushed productivity into every inch and corner of our time and lives. Part of this is driven by capitalistic, corporate culture. *Do more, climb the ladder, get more done with less, produce, produce, produce.*

The messaging is so pervasive that it extends far beyond our jobs and into our social, personal, and private lives. Combined with the constant buzzing of our phones, productivity culture urges us to log our progress and quantify our success publicly:

- Read at least two books a week to meet your 100 Goodreads goal.
- Log your workout times, glasses of water, steps.
- Be sure to keep up with the news.

- Track your social media interactions, analyse success.
- Don't forget to call your friends and make regular social plans.

There are even checklists for meditation!

None of these activities are inherently bad. Goals are important for all of us!

But the constant mental movement comes with a danger, too, because we can lose sight of what really matters. If we fill every nook and cranny of our minds with stimuli and goals and quantifiable markers of success, we leave our minds no room to breathe.

Our brains are remarkable things, capable of dreaming up better ways to be and express important essential ideas. Our brains are even capable of dreaming up new *ideals* and finding ways to make them into a reality. But without room to breathe, our minds never have room for their incredible potential.

Rediscovering The Value of Boredom

Boredom is often defined most by what it lacks—lack of stimulus, lack of engagement, lack of challenge. Sometimes it feels as though we are in a constant state of lacking, making it difficult to slow down—after all, our brains have been trained by contemporary culture to always seek attention, making that feeling of lack translate directly to anxiety. Most people find boredom to be an unpleasant sensation, preemptively going to great lengths to avoid feeling bored. In fact, one study found that that 67 percent of men and 25 percent of women would rather give themselves electric shocks than experience the boredom of sitting alone with their thoughts in an empty room.[3]

This is not to say that all kinds of boredom are positive. In some contexts, boredom can have negative effects. Jobs that require long periods of attentiveness within repetitive tasks—like security guards or air traffic controllers—can experience dangerous lapses in awareness. And boredom brought on by long-term social isolation has been linked to depression.[4] In some ways, it is understandable that our first instinct is to avoid boredom. But these are highly specific circumstances of boredom that are linked to other social dangers, namely repetitive motion and a lack of interpersonal connection. It was not until *very* recently that our culture and technology have allowed us to avoid boredom nearly entirely throughout our everyday lives, filling every second with content and engagement. Like overly repetitive tasks and social isolation, this state of constant stimulation is contrary to our natural state, in which some periods of boredom are not only natural but necessary. Recent research has shown that embracing more boredom can have enormous benefits to mental health.

The information age has created an environment overflowing with new and exciting content to engage with. Our attention has become a commodity in our modern era, and between work, advertising, and social content, there is great competition for our mental alertness. But our ability to give our focus to something is not without limits, and when it is stretched too thin, our brains become overloaded and stressed. When we try to give attention to everything, we give our true attention to nothing. Stepping away from input long enough to begin to feel bored can relieve that stress and give our brain time to allocate its attention resources more wisely and deliberately.

Allowing ourselves to be bored can also increase creativity and innovation. In her book *The Science of Boredom*, Sandi Mann reported a study that showed when people completed boring or engaging tasks without additional stimuli (no music playing, no other person to chat with, etc.), their wondering minds were able to come up with more creative solutions to problems and useful ideas. In the absence of external input, our imagination automatically engages and is allowed to create.[5]

This is because, while boredom can *feel* like a lacking state, in truth, it is a *searching* state. In a bored state, the engagement parts of our brain are at rest. As a result, this creative part of our brain looks for something new. Novelty-seeking is part of what makes humans adventurous and curious animals, which in turn drives our intelligence. Evolutionarily speaking, boredom is what led to the development of our frontal lobes, which increased our species' cognitive abilities including complex decision-making, risk assessment, and morality. The novelty drive also encourages new actions and exploration. Without boredom and the associated novelty drive, humans lose their ability to innovate. In fact, in his book, *The New Executive Brain*, Elkhonon Goldberg speculates that Christopher Columbus would never have left home if cell phones and Prozac prescriptions were available at the time.[6]

The trigger for novelty-seeking in boredom can feel inherently negative, emotionally. However, avoiding it entirely deprives us of our body's natural abilities and responses to it. As Andreas Elpidorou explains in his article for *Frontier Psychology*, boredom is an aversive state. He writes, "When one is bored, one is not content with one's situation. Boredom is one from which we seek to escape... If boredom is likened to an emotional trap, it is a trap that due to its own character fortunately 'pushes' us to escape from it." In this way, boredom is a crucial trigger emotion, motivating us to improve our situation. If we avoid it by numbing our brains with a constant flow of engaging but low-quality stimuli, we cut off our ability to seek out and take novel pleasure in new things that are closer to what is most important to us.

Certainly being bored can negatively affect our ability to focus, especially if what we are meant to focus on is the source of our boredom, as in the case of repetitive jobs. However, the solution is not to avoid boredom altogether. In fact, the negative effects of boredom on our brains are compounded when we do not learn to cope with periods of boredom. Seeking to *prevent* or limit boredom by switching to increasingly entertaining tasks actively weakens our mental ability to handle feelings of boredom. As a result, we become less and less able to use quiet states for creativity and motivation, much in the same way that a lack of use causes muscles to atrophy.[7]

Many psychologists have strongly recommended allowing children time to be bored, as this allows them to grow accustomed to the emotion. By making boredom a regular part of children's lives, they learn not only to tolerate a lack of external stimulation, but also to use their internal resources to tap into innate creativity.[8] Learning this skill at a young age is one of the best paths to emotional maturity and self-control as adults.

The Connection Between Boredom and Sleep

While there are benefits to boredom, more research is needed to fully understand the role of boredom in our brains and the limits of its positive influence. After all, it was not long ago that people considered sleep as a lacking state and did not understand why it was necessary. We only knew the negative effects of too little sleep.

We now know that sleep is far from a state of idleness for our brains. While we sleep, our brains are consumed with crucial tasks, even if those tasks do not require our conscious attention. In his book *Why We Sleep*, Matthew Walker outlines our brains' incredible processes during sleep, explaining why sufficient sleep is essential to our health and well-being, both physical and mental. Sleep regulates blood sugar, metabolism, muscle condition, and cellular regeneration. The cognitive benefits of good sleep include improved memory and mental acuity; improved motor skills, "muscle memory" and proficiency; and improved creativity.[9] While we sleep, especially in the rapid eye movement (REM) stages of sleep, our brains sort through memories of the previous day, discarding unnecessary recollections and making connections to previous memories. In this way, the brain categorizes our memories in a passive state of learning that is essential, despite our unconsciousness throughout the process. Recent research has even shown that the brain washes itself of cell-damaging plaque and toxins during sleep, improving neural connectivity and effectively preventing a range of neurological disorders.[10] It is increasingly clear that sleep is far from a "lacking" state, and the same may prove true for boredom as well.

Given the benefits of boredom to creativity and

problem solving, it seems logical that boredom serves a similar brain function as sleep. Halting the constant flow of input for a while gives the brain both the space and the motivation to go to work on what it has already collected. Previous observations and thoughts can be pulled out, dusted off, and put together in new and enlightening ways.

Periods of boredom, especially in the late evening, can also improve the quality of rest, making our brain's sleep functions even more effective. While excessive boredom throughout waking hours can negatively impact sleep, intentionally removing stimuli in the evenings to trigger a bored state can make the transition from waking to sleeping easier and more pleasant, resulting in deeper, more effective sleep and rest.

When Food Feels Boring

When first transitioning into a diet based on meals made with few, whole ingredients, our first instinct may be to consider this "boring" food.

However, it is important to remember what the abundance of over-engineered food has done to our ability to feel sated. The bliss point engineering of food has blasted our palate's ability to appreciate simplicity and detect nuance, especially in fresh food. Essentially, our food culture has trained our palate to need an explosion of powerful flavours and immediate pleasure sensations from fat and sugar in order to feel that we are eating something good.

So to change our palates as well as our habits, we must learn to be okay with being bored with our food—at least at first.

Just as being in nature and practising deliberate boredom can make us more creative and sensitive to the beauty around us, eating whole, simple foods consistently gradually increase our appreciation for them. We can apply those creative ideas to different combinations of spices and healthy flavourings. We can learn to appreciate the difference between a grass-fed and finished steak and a factory-bred one or the difference between early spring asparagus and mid-summer asparagus.

As I see in every client I work with, you will begin to experience what it is like to truly feel better. Over time, as your body runs on food that truly nourishes it, it will regain its natural equilibrium. Paired with deliberate mental boredom, that equilibrium will allow you to feel better, think more clearly, and enjoy more of your every moment of life.

Deliberate Boredom

If you've ever solved a difficult problem while washing your hair, you can understand the importance of giving your brain time away from stimuli. The problem is that many of us *only* give our brains time away from stimulation while we are in the shower. So many of us have been caught up in the drive to fill every moment of our lives with productivity that our minds fill with guilt the moment our attention begins to wander without purpose.

To break that pattern, we need to make boredom purposeful. We do this by deliberately making space for boredom in our lives. We hear too much about the "time we cannot get back," and that should apply to uncommitted time as well.

One important caveat is worth mentioning here.

Although we want to make boredom purposeful, we do *not* want to add it to our growing daily to-do list. Do not time your boredom, and for goodness' sake, do not add boredom to your calendar. The state of being bored is just that—a state—it should not become another item for you to frown on at the end of the day, wondering whether you truly achieved the task of boredom.

Instead, we can all look for little pockets, finding room for boredom in our daily lives by giving ourselves space for it. When you're driving in your car, occasionally turn the sound off and listen to nothing. Let your mind wander and give your brain space to fill the few minutes with whatever thoughts come to mind.

Try not to schedule things so closely that you have no time to walk around aimlessly. After work, give yourself a buffer of ten or fifteen minutes with no expectations or tasks to complete. And, of course, step away from your phone.

Our lives are often so noisy that it can be hard to find those moments that allow us to make boredom a positive habit. The longer we go between periods of purposeful boredom, the harder it can be to sit in the feeling without the overpowering urge to pick up our phones and scroll or jump up off the couch to find some household tasks or another.

One way to ease into and make time for the feeling is to seek a connection with nature. Spending time in nature while we leave behind phones, to-do lists, and tasks can help us get connected to our Paleolithic forebears, even if only in short bursts. I recommend a minimum of thirty minutes, three times per week to start. (This, at least, is something you *can* put on your calendar if you absolutely must.)

Sit in nature—it does not have to be wilderness, as any quiet, green space will do—without your phone or any other tools you would usually reach for to fill idle time. This can ease you into a state of boredom gently. The boredom produced by an empty room, or a monotonous task can feel closest to a form of torture, but that form of boredom is not usually associated with being and among the ambient life of nature. After all, there are stimuli in nature—birdsong, the textures of grass and wind, and the brilliant range of natural colours. But usually—at least in the safe, quiet spaces we are most likely to visit—these stimuli require very little from us. They do not beg for a response in the way our phones do. Unlike social media alerts, the bees' buzz is gentle and calming.

Outdoors writer Alex Roddie reflects in his personal blog that boredom is impossible in nature—at least when it comes to that torturous, modern brand of boredom. He notes that our ancestors "lived more vital lives, closer to the nature around them and the nature of their own selves. Today, Boredom and stress seem like two sides of the same coin, chasing our fragmented attention like snakes."[11] In nature, we use all our senses to take in the environment. If we are open to it with nothing to pull us back to a productivity-mindset, that environment can soothe all the negative feelings that we associate with boredom, allowing our brains to reap the benefits.

Intuitive Guidance

Understanding that boredom, like most things, can have negative effects in particular contexts and amounts, it is important that we use our intuition to approach boredom in moderation the same way we use our intuition to eat appropriate amounts of food. The goal of intuitive eating is never to *prevent* the negative feeling of hunger, nor is it to prolong the sensation of hunger as long as possible, but to wait for that bodily sensation as a signal that it is time to eat.

We must treat the balance between attention and boredom the same way. By never allowing boredom to arise, we are depleting our attention and over-consuming engagement. Our over-saturated brains lose the creative ability to innovate, self-regulate, and re-focus on what really matters to us. By purposefully embracing boredom, we unlock the full power of our minds. We accept the quiet, boring moments because we realise that they are far preferable to noisy, overwhelming lives.

9

COLLECTIVE FOOD

ROUGHLY TEN THOUSAND YEARS AGO, civilizations began to settle around riverbanks—the Amazon, the Nile, the Mississippi, the Indus, and the Yangtze. Permanent agricultural centres began to grow and were tended by growing communities of people. Leadership and structures of the hierarchy formed to organize this labour. Alongside this major advancement for mankind came an insidious caveat. As leaders grew more and more disconnected from the production of the community's food, access to quality food grew lopsided. The lowest people on the hierarchy were relegated to food that could be produced quickly and superficially fill the belly—grains and grasses. Rare and more precious foods were reserved for the leadership. Over the millennium, this gap has only widened.

With the technology and the knowledge we have today, we would appear as gods to early man. And yet, we have not applied that innovation to closing the inequality gap, which is still perhaps most pronounced in our access to nutritious food.

Global Food Insecurity and Nutritional Inequity

The World Food Programme (WFP) categorizes populations by a 5-stage rating called IPC, or Integrated Food Security Phase Classification.[1] Phase 1 indicates little to no food insecurity. Phase 2, Stressed, indicates populations that have to make difficult choices in order to fulfill their nutritional needs. Phase 3, Crisis, indicates populations that experience significant gaps in food consumption, leading to malnutrition, or are only able to meet minimal food needs by sacrificing essential assets. Phase 4, Emergency, describes populations who face large food consumption gaps resulting in acute malnutrition and excess mortality or extreme loss of assets that will lead to future food consumption gaps. Phase 5, Catastrophe, indicates populations that are blighted, have little or no access to edible food, and face imminent starvation.[2]

Between 4.5 and 5 billion people—the majority of the planet—live in Phase 1, but this leaves nearly two billion people in a state of stress surrounding getting adequate calories to sustain themselves. The populations in Crisis and Emergency stages have been growing rapidly since the turn of the century, and recent escalations in conflict zones have put new populations in true catastrophic famine conditions. The populations most in danger include areas like sub-Saharan Africa, which has been most affected by climate shocks that decimate their local production. Areas that are in sustained states of conflict like Ukraine, Yemen, Syria, the West Bank, and Afghanistan face the direst Phases of 4 and 5.

The WFP does essential and life-saving work in helping these populations, with a focus on populations in Phase 3 or greater. They provide direct food aid including both ration and cash support. They are a leader in logistics and supply chain management, often acting as the logistical arm of the United Nations during emergencies. They manage the storage, transportation, and delivery of food and other essential supplies. They face great obstacles to their work including redirections of their funding, supply chain disruptions due to COVID-19, climate change, and conflict, as well as the bureaucratic and logistical difficulties inherent in running operations in over eighty countries.[3]

The WFP needs continued support because starvation is a global crisis that cannot be addressed without sustained and increased aid, but these categorizations are insufficient to truly depict the scope of the problem of food inequity. That is because these measures only account for critical, immediate danger from lack of any form of nutrition. It does not attempt to measure the *quality* of the nutrition at any level.

The 2022 Global Nutrition Report (GNR) emphasizes the need to have a bigger picture understanding of nutritional needs when making both global and local efforts to combat poor nutrition, hunger, and disease. The report refers to the "double burden of nutrition—two sides of one crisis" that "has vast health, economic, and environmental implications, affecting every country of the world in some form."[4]

The problem is that under nutrition is only one branch of malnutrition. Diet-related non-communicable diseases (NCDs), mainly obesity, diabetes, cardiovascular disease, and cancer also contribute to the global malnutrition crisis and cause suffering and increased mortality in populations all over the world. The GNR identifies markers of malnutrition in both children and adults. In children under five, it measures wasting, stunting, obesity, and anaemia. In adults, it tracks key NCD indicators like salt intake, blood pressure, and diabetes. In 2022, nearly all the GNR indicators of health were determined to be "off course," indicating they were falling well below the goals needed to slow and reverse growing trends of these mortality causes by 2030.[5]

While millions face the desperate need for food, any food, billions more struggle to fully meet their nutritional needs with the product most available to them. The 1.5 billion people in Phase 2 of food insecurity are not immediate aid targets of organizations like the WFP but are still in dire need of help. They are regulated to the cheapest sources of food available to them, and that is most commonly the ultra-processed, grain-based foods pushed most by profit-led food manufacturers. These foods are the likely cause of growing rates of NCDs in developed countries with a wide internal income disparity. As noted by Derek Headey:

"The high cost of many nutrient-dense foods in populations most at risk of undernutrition is a major barrier to resolving undernutrition and warrants urgent policy attention. A key objective of pro-equity, nutrition-sensitive food policies should be to improve the affordability of nutrient-rich foods, both economy-wide and for the poorest households... At the level of a whole economy, this could be done by achieving lower prices through improved agricultural and trade policies."[6]

To address this, global efforts to improve malnutrition must work to increase the local and global diversity of crops and work to lower the cost and widen the availability of nutritious food across political and economic borders.

The Influence of Big Food and Big Grain

Global efforts to address nutrition gaps have long recognized the importance of changing agricultural practices but are stymied by profit-driven corporations that throw their weight around in order to maintain the status quo that benefits their bottom lines. This is the "Big Food" model.

"Big Food" refers to large multinational corporations that dominate the food and beverage industry through their extensive market reach, influence on consumer habits, and significant control over agricultural production and supply chains. These companies, including Nestle, Pepsi and Coca-Cola, Unilever, Kraft, Mondalez, and General Mills, as well as dozens of subdivisions, have vast product portfolios, global operations, and considerable economic and political power. The control of the market by these companies can be seen on our grocery store shelves, but their influence does not stop there. Given their massive scale, these companies also have a huge influence over our macro-economic systems.

As I outlined in Chapter 1, the products these companies produce are designed for their addictive qualities, and on the scale of Big Food, this creates a massive and inflated demand for the raw materials that go into these products. To meet this demand, "Big Agricultural" companies have in turn promoted monoculture farming, dedicating these huge tracks of land to single crops like wheat and corn. In turn, Big Agriculture pressured meat manufacturers to shift their practices to rely heavily on their excess crops to sustain CAFOs. Together, these three monoliths—food manufacturing, agriculture, and meat—have collaborated to pressure governments around the world to institute policies to support these practices. The US subsidizes crops like corn, wheat, and soybeans. International trade is pressured to prioritize the export of these foods, first by growing so large and interconnected that multiple economies rely on them, and then by pointing to that reliance as evidence that their business must be the priority of every logistical and supply chain consideration. Smaller manufacturers and farmholders are also subject to these structures, as the path to ethical, sustainable farming is obstructed by the prevalence of these poor practices and the structures that hold them up.

The system is so large and interconnected that disruption of grain production and exportation in a single country like Ukraine is felt in every country in the world —whether in the rise of food prices or in shortages.

Because these massive structures built by Big Food are in place, altruistic efforts and funding are also subject to over-dependence on grains. Prabhu Pingali notes for the GNR that research and development funding typically focus on our culture's most overused and abused foods—grains, grasses, and other foods that are often considered the basic building blocks of our food supply despite their low nutritional value.[7] As Pingali explains, this global focus on grains has only shifted the problem of food insecurity, rather than alleviating it. Due to both international export policies and humanitarian intervention, total calorie consumption has risen over the past three decades, especially in countries that were categorized as Phases 3 and 4 populations in the 1980s. However, this has not solved the problem of micronutrient malnutrition, which is the primary cause of stunting in children worldwide.

Stunting is a condition that arises from chronic

malnutrition during the most critical periods of growth and development in early life, particularly in the first thousand days which is from conception until the age of two. Stunting leads to lifelong issues like impaired growth, delayed cognitive development, weakened immune systems, and increased risk of chronic disease. Cases of stunting have increased even as caloric consumption has superficially changed the status of many populations from Crisis to Stressed. In some areas, there are growing populations of individuals who will experience *both* stunting *and* obesity in their lifetimes. To provide not just food, but health, strength, and longevity, agricultural practices must shift. As Pingali concludes, "A holistic view of agricultural policy would require governments to look beyond the major staples to ensure availability of and access to a wider and healthier basket of food."[8]

This is also an economic issue. *The Economist* has examined the causes and effects of climate shocks and rising conflicts on the global food markets and recommends significant shifts. First, they recommend diversification—both in the products grown and the origins of products, and second, they recommend that nations invest in their own food security by growing their own agricultural practices. In 2022, the World Bank announced that thirty billion dollars would be made available to help countries become more food secure.[9]

While *The Economist* emphasizes that true nation-by-nation self-sufficiency may not be truly possible, increased efforts toward that can help lessen the devastating impacts of climate shocks and conflicts that are felt reverberating throughout the global supply chain. This can also help disrupt the overwhelming influence of corporate heavyweights in the market, providing space for more research and development in sustainable, local farming practices.

Pathways to Sustainable Practices: Big and Small

For over seventy-five years, there have been increasing calls for more sustainable farming practices. Existing agricultural practices like monoculture farming, excessive irrigation, aggressive pesticides and fertilizers, and soil impaction have led to nutrient depletion in the soil over time. When land has been so mistreated that it becomes desert-like and cannot support animal or plant life, it is deemed "desertified."

Combined with urban growth, it is estimated that approximately 24 percent of the world's landmass has been degraded.[10] Over 1.9 billion hectares (over seven million square miles) of previously farmable land has been desertified. Africa is most severely affected, with 65 percent of its agricultural land becoming unusable and the Sahara Desert expanding its borders each year. In China, the Gobi is also expanding, with 27 percent of land determined to be desertified since the mid-20th century.[11] This has increased the reliance on international food imports, which further increases the need for shelf-stable, often less nutritious foods. This reliance also increases the power and influence of massive international corporations. These corporations are not motivated to change agricultural practices and policies when doing so would threaten their own monopoly.

It was long theorized that increased animal farming was to blame for blighted land, from overgrazing to the strain from producing ample animal feed. Many areas tried to improve land conditions by reducing land used for animal farming. However, this proved to be misguided, not only because we need animal production and farming for adequate nutrition, but because the effects on the land were nowhere near as beneficial as presumed. New ideas were needed, and Allan Savory developed a different strategy—one that, if imitated around the world, could help both heal the land and make individual nations more self-sufficient and food secure.

Allan Savory is a Zimbabwean ecologist, livestock farmer, and environmentalist. His new idea for agriculture became known as Holistic Management. In the 1960s, he worked as a game ranger in what was then Rhodesia.[12] Observing the widespread desertification and degradation of the land, he also initially believed that reducing animal numbers was the key to reversing these trends. However, his early efforts in wildlife management led to disappointing results, prompting a fundamental reevaluation of his assumptions.

Savory came to what was then a controversial conclusion: livestock, if managed correctly, could be used to heal the land. He proposed that by mimicking the natural grazing patterns of wild herbivores, livestock could help restore degraded grasslands.[13] This insight laid the groundwork for Holistic Management, a framework that considers the interconnectedness of environmental, economic, and social factors in land management decisions.

Holistic Management promotes the use of planned grazing, where livestock are moved frequently across pastures in a way that prevents overgrazing and allows vegetation to recover.[14] This method aims to enhance soil health, increase biodiversity, and sequester carbon, contributing to both sustainable agriculture and climate change mitigation. The approach also emphasizes decision-making that considers the complexity of ecosystems, striving for solutions that are beneficial for both the land and the people who depend on it.

Savory's Holistic Management plan is based on four key insights into our relationship with nature as organized farmers.[15]

The first key insight is that "Nature functions in wholes." This philosophy emphasizes that nature is a whole that is greater than a sum of its parts. Savory argues, "Not only is the world more complex than we understand, but it's more complex than we can EVER understand . . . Individual parts do not exist in nature, only wholes, and these form and shape each other." In other words, we cannot remove any part of nature and expect our environment to function in the same way. It is a powerful reminder that we cannot simply isolate a piece of land and use it indefinitely as a food-producing tract because natural growth is influenced by everything around it.

The second key insight is that agricultural land is not the same everywhere, and any plan must be adapted to both its current state and its natural state prior to human interference. Savory adapted the "brittleness" scale which ranges from 1 (evergreen tropical forest) to 10 (true desert) based on how well humidity is distributed throughout the year, and how quickly dead vegetation breaks down. Understanding land's place on the brittleness scale can determine what the healing process can look like and what methods will be effective.

The third key insight is understanding the predator-prey connection to land health. In Africa, Savory had taken note of how herds of game animals behaved in the wild, especially in the presence of active predators. They would bunch together for safety, trampling plants, breaking up the soil, and covering areas with concentrated patches of dung and urine before moving on when the predator left the area. This proved to be not only good for the land, but vital for areas of more brittle environments. Savory realised that by managing livestock in a way that mimics the behaviour produced by the predator-prey relationship, we could begin to restore the brittle African grasslands, and that similar adoptions would have positive effects in less brittle areas as well.

The fourth key insight reveals the common misconception that land destruction was caused by too many animals, prompting virtually all land-improvement schemes to call for the reduction or removal of animals. The supposed causation didn't hold up to scrutiny, because if herding animals blighted land, why then were areas like the American Plains so much healthier during the hundreds of years when they hosted the largest herds of grazing animals in the world? The answer came by examining the natural behaviour of grazing animals, which are nomadic in nature, never occupying the same patch of land for too long. Grazing is a necessary part of the soil cycle, and it only becomes harmful *overgrazing* when animals are not permitted to move from place to place as they would naturally.

Mimicking the natural behaviour of herding or prey animals according to the various environments allows for the soil to maintain its health and stay productive.[16]

With these insights, Holistic Management has been healing and bringing back land on the brink of becoming a permanent desert in various places around the world, including Canada, South America, and Africa.

Expanding these practices around the globe will continue to heal the land, provide a pathway for more self-sufficiency for individual nations, and potentially break up the monopoly on practices that Big Food and Big Agriculture have enjoyed for far too long.

Collective Action for Our Collective Food

Our modern food industry has shifted our food focus to profit margins over health, which affects the global environment and the efficiency of aid efforts, since aid resources are also limited by what is being manufactured. These tactics hurt everyone in every category of food security. Big Food knows this but will do nothing if it means hurting their bottom line.

For better or for worse, our local and global communities are intertwined and interlocked. I wish I had a simple, quick solution—or even a quick, complicated one—for dismantling these systems that are making us all sicker and sicker. They were built over the course of several generations, and very likely the problem will take generations to completely reverse.

But the interlocked nature of our communities goes both ways.

What we do, for our families and for our local communities, can be felt on a macro level if we all act collectively to demand the change that we want to see in the world. We must think about our food as the link in the chains that connect us all to one another and the environment. This is the only way to save our own health, the health of our community, and the health of our planet.

One small action we can take to help with the global burden of processed foods on our health and land is to support our small local farmers who are actively trying to regenerate the land and work with nature, while producing healthy whole foods. Once we become aware of the problem, through reading this book, each of us can make small changes in how we purchase our food. Given our collective purchase power, these are changes that would have a large-scale impact on the stranglehold on Big Food.

"Never doubt that a small group of thoughtful committed individuals can change the world. In fact, it's the only thing that ever has."
MARGARET MEAD

10

ALL IN YOUR HEAD

THE MORE I progress in my own journey, aligning my actions to my values and finding better ways to safeguard my health through nutrition, the more I treasure my time in nature. The quiet and ease of nature provides peace like nothing else can. The green space I visit most frequently is my garden.

I am not particularly ambitious about my garden—it is made up of small, three-by-four-foot vegetable beds—but even that little space provides plenty of seasonal vegetables for my family's table and an opportunity for me to better understand how plants grow, what makes healthy soil, and have a deeper understanding of how food is grown. It may not be huge or elaborate, but when I work in the black dirt, I think about the billions of microscopic but essential organisms and nutrients hidden there. When you touch black dirt on a cloudy day, you can still feel the warmth of yesterday's sun. Under the harsh, arid light of midsummer, you can feel the cool moisture from the previous rain, still kept in balance in the earth. I am far from an expert gardener, but coaxing a delicious crown of broccoli or a deeply vibrant spray of kale helps me connect to the natural way things grow. The fat, furry bumblebees busy at their collective work remind me of how everything in the universe is deeply interconnected. It helps me to feel centred, and it nurtures my sense of awe for nature, our planet, and the amazing abundance it provides for us.

Growth does not happen all at once, but with patience and care, it happens inevitably. The seed bursts and the first radicle pushes down into the earth, pulling in moisture and nutrients. Stems tunnel up into the air and leaves unfurl under the sun to best catch its light. Cells divide and multiply and the plant expands, because growing is at the heart of nature.

We grow too, even well beyond adulthood when so many of us believe we should have everything figured out. Our minds, abilities, and influence can keep growing and improving as long as we provide the space for ourselves to do so.

Making Health Central to Our Values and Identity

Our values are central to who we are and our identities, both in our communities and in our own self-perception. Sometimes, these values are inherited from our culture or family or religious beliefs. However, we can and should make deliberate choices about what matters to us and let those values be our guiding light in all our decisions and efforts.

When we choose our touchstone values, health—our own, our family's, our community's, and our planet's—can be a powerful focus to improve our lives both singly and collectively.

But as a value, health can also be fraught with difficulty and tension.

Choosing to value your health means you will need to say no to things, most often in a social context. Saying no can be difficult, not only because of personal temptation but because we naturally want to avoid hurting or offending others by not joining in what they are doing. However, over time, compromising your values causes stress, anxiety, and mental anguish. That stress can have massive long-term impacts on our lives—it is simply too high a price to pay for avoiding the discomfort of social friction in the moment. Living your values is a matter of practice. When you do your best to practice living according to your health, it becomes easier over time.

Aligning your life with your values despite others' reluctance to do so not only fosters consistency and motivation, it also enriches your journey toward health and happiness. Recognizing the importance of this connection empowers us to make choices that truly resonate with who we are and what we value most.

Adopting a Mindset Framework

In her book, *Mindset: The New Psychology of Success*, Carol Dweck outlines two fundamental frameworks of how we think about ourselves and our identities.[1] Either framework will have a massive influence over our actions and how successful we are at pursuing goals, but one offers opportunity while the other mires us in stagnation.

She calls these two opposite frameworks a "fixed" mindset and a "growth" mindset.

Those who hold a primarily fixed mindset believe, consciously or unconsciously, that there is a built-in cap on their success and that this pinnacle is determined by their core identity. For instance, those in a fixed mindset may put significant emphasis on IQ as a predetermined marker of intelligence. If they learn that they have a high IQ at a young age, the idea that they are intelligent will integrate seamlessly into their identities. They will seek to prove their natural cognitive ability over and over because it is who they are, but they will not seek to expand their intelligence, as they do not believe it is possible.

In this mindset, individuals make choices in reaction to these supposed "fixed points." Those in a fixed mindset avoid risking failure as much as possible. They are afraid of hitting that cap and experiencing the disappointment of reaching their hard limit, because they erroneously believe that it would reveal an indelible flaw in their character. So they avoid testing their "limits." Those who learn to identify themselves as "bad at math," for example, will choose careers in areas that do not require skill with numbers, avoiding the risk of failure.

Those with a growth mindset do not believe in any inherent and immutable limit to their capabilities—they focus only on the obstacles and shortfalls they *currently* have, which can be overcome.

When it comes to the questions of intelligence and skill, psychology supports the framework of the growth mindset.

Returning to the example of the IQ test, psychologists have been reducing their reliance on these tests for decades because they are not as accurate a measure of intelligence as once assumed. The test is overly narrow in scope and subject to a great deal of cultural bias, but most importantly, IQ tests provide a static measure of intelligence, not accounting for growth or changes over time.

Intelligence is dynamic and can be influenced by various factors, including environment, education, and personal experiences. Psychologists are increasingly adopting holistic approaches to assessment, considering a wide range of factors that contribute to individuals' cognitive and emotional functioning. This includes qualitative assessments, observations, and alternative testing methods. Neurologically, IQ testing is also severely limited. Advances in neuroscience have highlighted the complexity of intelligence and moved away from the static measure of IQ scores.

The brain is not determined by a set and static "quotient" of anything, and that includes our intelligence. On the contrary, our brains are like muscles. The more we challenge ourselves, the stronger our capacity for thought.

We understand this instinctively when it comes to children—no one would assume that a two-year-old is just bad at language and always will be. But as we age, a fixed mindset can develop and give us false impressions of the nature of our brains and abilities. We can continue to learn throughout our lifetimes. Each time we learn something, new connections form in our brains. With each new connection, a new pair of neurons learn to communicate through synapses, and our ability to think multiples. Eventually, the process becomes exponential, with new connections forming to make cognitive tasks easier and more efficient. Things that once felt impossible, like a new language or technical skill, can become second nature over time. The only true "limits" to our brains' abilities are the time and effort we put into our growth.

What is so compelling about Dr. Dweck's research is our power to shift our mindsets. When we know growth is possible, we are more likely to push ourselves. In a study working with adolescents, students were given academic support through a series of small group or one-on-one tutoring sessions across several subjects. Every student was provided with the same support, but a portion of students received an additional workshop in mindset in which they learned to shift their self-understanding and identities. The goal of this workshop was to help students realise not only that improvement was possible, but that growth is a natural outcome of effort and hard work. The study found that those who took the mindset workshop improved more quickly—and more overall—than those who did not. Most of the students who did not participate in the mindset workshop showed little or no improvement in their grades. Reports from the classroom teachers, who did not know who was enrolled in the mindset workshop, frequently reported that enrolled students were voluntarily increasing their individual efforts. They asked for help both in class and in their free periods. They requested opportunities to try again on assignments and scored better the second time. They became active participants in their education, and that led to immediate improvement in their skills.

The students in Dr. Dweck's study show that those who can shift to a growth mindset are also more likely to ask for help because they believe that their problems are surmountable and therefore help is valuable. Those students who received tutoring but not the mindset workshop did not understand that their improvement was possible. Therefore, the academic help they received was much less effective. As Dr. Dweck concludes, "The mindset workshop put students in charge of their brains. Freed from the vise of the fixed mindset, [the students] could now use their minds more freely and fully."[2]

The two mindsets have very different attitudes when it comes to hard work, failure and success. Those in a fixed mindset shy away from truly difficult and novel challenges because having to work hard may prove that they do not "have what it takes." Those in a growth mindset come to love hard work for the new abilities and skills it helps them acquire. Those in a fixed mindset see failure as something that will permanently define them. They believe that once you *fail* you *are a failure.* Those in a growth mindset understand that failure is not something you "are" but something you experience. Failure is not pleasant, and it is certainly not as satisfying as success, but it is not integrated into their personal identities.

The different attitude toward success is perhaps the most telling and key distinction. Those in a fixed mindset think of success as an *end point,* something that one is either entitled to or not entitled to, based on their identity. For those in a growth mindset, there is no endpoint. Success represents only a forward momentum.

In a fixed mindset, you will give yourself credit for doing things that came to you naturally and easily. This will feel like validation for *who you are.* In a growth mindset, things that are easy to do offer very little, because you only attain growth through challenge—by stretching your abilities further than what you have already proven yourself capable of.

In other words, if you believe you are static, you will be static. Your inertia will keep you rooted and unchanging, and you will continue to feel the pain of the gap between who you would like to be and who you are.

If you *know* you can *grow,* your efforts are more likely to become gains and give you that momentum you need to keep them. By shifting your mindset, you can fall in love with growth itself.

The Trap of Moderation

Balance is important to maintaining health and well-being. We must balance work and rest, stimulation and boredom, reflection and creativity—these are all things that must work together in healthy cycles.

However, sometimes a search for balance—especially in a diet—can be an excuse that keeps us trapped by preventing us from breaking out of bad habits. The most common way this shows up in my clients' lives is through the advice to eat everything in moderation. It sounds sensible, even kind because it makes no hard and fast rules nor all-encompassing judgments about any particular foods.

But this advice often leads us down a path that is neither sustainable nor aligned with our long-term health goals.

What we consume in moderation tends to creep up gradually over time, such that we may not even notice it. A glass of wine a day becomes two; a sugary treat in the mid-afternoon becomes one in mid-morning, one in mid-afternoon, and maybe a couple in the evening. Soon, our consumption is far from "moderate," and with the addictive qualities of the foods we tend to eat in "moderation," we are soon trapped in a cycle that makes it very difficult to reduce our intake back to those little allowances here and there. This is the nature of addictive substances.

Those who urge moderation often cite the maxim that *the dose makes the poison*, meaning that our bodies can often handle unhealthful substances in infrequent small doses. But of course those unhealthful substances are still unhealthful—just because we limit them to small amounts does not mean that they are *good for us.*

For example, previous studies that posited the health benefits of regular, small amounts of red wine have been discredited by more recent research. In 2023, the World Health Organization declared unequivocally that no amount of alcohol is safe. Any previously cited benefits to heart health are significantly outweighed by the risks and ill effects of alcohol.[3]

Just because your body *can* process something does not mean that it *should.*

Moderation was not a concept our ancestors considered. They were focused on survival, and the most efficient way to survive with the fewest calories and most nutrients was through meat consumption. When they came upon fruit, honey, or vegetables, they did not scoff. They simply tried to figure out how best to consume them.

But they did not have big business muddying the waters. When they came upon grasses that the ruminants consumed, they were not told to eat them in moderation or as "part of a balanced diet." Instead, they had to consider the work involved in transforming grasses and grains into bread. This level of processing would likely require more calories and other resources than the food could eventually provide.

Today we say moderation means a balanced approach to nutrition; however, this can be a slippery slope. We have used "moderation" as a reason to consume foods that work against the human genome, leading to digestive and microbiome disruption and chronic illness, all in the name of balance.

Do Not Wait Upon Wealth to Prioritize Your Health

Becoming financially secure is a goal for everyone not just because money gives us the ability to buy *stuff*. It is also a goal because it represents a level of freedom and ease. All too often, I see hard-working people who put their health aside by assuming that only the wealthy have the time and resources to prioritize their health.

In many ways, this is a symptom of a fixed mindset. *If I were wealthy, I could focus on my health and align my life with my values. Since I am not, I cannot.*

This is faulty logic!

As we have explored throughout this book, healthy choices are not limited by dollar amounts, but by effort and commitment. When you are committed to growth and aligning your choices and identity with your core values, you can and will find ways to improve your health on any budget. Simple meals made with whole foods and few ingredients are attainable with just a little planning and practice. Movement and consistent exercise do not need to cost anything but time. Nothing could possibly cost *less* than allowing room for boredom in your daily life.

Truthfully, regardless of our income status, we cannot afford *not* to prioritize our health. It is the single most essential component to our happiness and well-being. And in our modern world, chronic illnesses are diseases connected to lifestyle, not genetics.

If, while reading this book, you have found yourself thinking, *That would be nice if I could afford to,* or *That would be nice if I had the time,* or *That would be nice, but first I have to (insert other obligation here),* I invite you to reflect carefully on your mindset. Are those obstacles really fixed, or do you just *feel* that they are? If you accepted that the changes you want to make in your life are possible, starting right now, what would your first move be?

All the information, new perspectives, and advice throughout this book might seem daunting. So many aspects of our modern life push against us, making it feel impossible to change. There are the big-picture obstacles of greedy corporate interests and misguided governmental policies that create systems that work against our collective health. There is an entire, well-meaning culture surrounding food and body image that can take us down destructive paths. Then on a micro level, we have the inertia of our habits, the addictions that have built up over time, and the onslaught of stimuli from our modern world that make it so hard just to *think* and *be* and *enjoy*.

Together, these obstacles can feel like insurmountable opposition to change.

But with a shift of our mindsets, all the things that work against us can be seen, not as impenetrable barriers, but as a series of opportunities to become better, stronger, and more aligned with our values. We never have to accept the status quo as a hard-set limit to who we are.

When we face challenges and meet them, the gains we have made stay with us, whether through acquiring a new skill at work, meeting a benchmark in our fitness goals, or overcoming one of our poor habits and replacing it with a healthier one. We can then take that win and apply that energy to the next gain, and the next. In this way, our gains ripple out and what seemed once to be daunting challenges become exciting opportunities to keep testing ourselves and growing.

The same is true for us all, collectively. When we live

according to our values through our spending and working choices—and support others to do the same—those social gains stay with us, too.

To accept the status quo as a limit is to languish.

It can get better. *We* can be better.

AFTERWORD

Castrignano D'ei Greci, Italy is 4,746 miles away from Oakville, Ontario, Canada.

Half a world, it seems, separates my life from that little farming village where my grandmother grew up picking dandelions and stealing from the edges of farms.

The farms of Castrignano D'ei Greci are supported by the fertile calcareous soils that nurture lush olive groves and vineyards, their roots reaching deep into the earth's limestone. Meanwhile, Oakville, Ontario, is graced by the legacy of ancient glaciers, dotted with flourishes of sandy and clay loam soils. Though separated by oceans and miles, the lands share a common tale of Earth's bounty.

Though the soils and the climates are very different, the processes of life are the same—the seeds sprout and grow, blossoms open at the end of their stems, the insects pollinate, and the animals eat. The vital chemicals of life are passed along, reformed and remixed and used to create new generations of life in an endless cycle.

When I can spend time in nature, those thousands of

miles seem to mean very little, because I realise that we are so closely connected. My grandmother feels close because I know she occupies a place in the cycle, just as I do. Just as we all do. That connection goes back through the generations. For thousands and thousands of years, we have all been a part of something so much larger than ourselves, consuming and reproducing, learning and passing along what we have learned through our words and our very genes.

Honouring Our Ancestral Connection

It is no wonder that cultural practices all around the world centre on shared meals, because eating is the most intimate part of that connection to our lineage, as we quite literally take in what the earth offers to continue and enrich our lives. We should honour that connection by eating with consideration and intention.

Eating whole and simple foods has led me to a greater feeling of connection with my ancestors and with nature.

Doing so, for both me and my family, has come with the added benefits of curing our stomach ailments, regulating and maintaining a comfortable weight, improved hormonal health, and an overall improved feeling of wellness and strength.

Throughout my journey of redefining my relationship to food, I have endeavoured to find out why this is so important. The answers taught me the crucial role of understanding how our bodies work and how they use food. With this book I have attempted to share many of the big lessons I have learned along the way, both about individual health and the deep-rooted sickness in our global food markets and systems.

I hope these pages have inspired you to examine your own relationship with food and wellness.

As connected as we are, we are all different, so your own health and wellness journey may not look exactly like mine or anyone else's. Our modern world is extraordinarily complicated with pressures on what we eat ranging from trillion-dollar global economies down to social judgment around the office snack table.

And of course, there is our own inertia to overcome—ingrained habits and addictions that we might not even be aware we have.

There are enormous obstacles to change, both for each of us individually and collectively as a society.

But change is possible.

On my own journey and through my work as a nutritionist, I have learned that transformation requires support. I embarked on my own journey with the support of my husband and family, even though we did not always see eye to eye. In my practice, I offer similarly uplifting support for my clients, and I find so much joy in their growth toward greater health and wellness. Every client I have worked with has been a little different, so my approach has always been to tailor my experience, training, and expertise to what will serve them best during our time together.

But there is one constant in this work: a common goal to intentionally program a new mindset that is built on each client's personal values system. I find that if we work with this intention in mind, we can set goals based on our value standards making us much more likely to succeed.

Most of what we learn, both consciously and unconsciously, comes from our environment and childhood upbringing. We have very little say in this experience.

The first step for all of us is deciding that *we* are the designers of our own lives. That we will design a life so we can live in alignment and harmony with what we believe in. So that we can honour what matters most to us.

This does not happen like the flip of a switch. This type of holistic transformation takes time, energy, and patience.

Be kind to yourself on this journey and understand that it takes sustained intention to shake off our old habits, overcome bad influence, and unlearn harmful advice. You are redesigning your life. Few things are more worthy of hard work and determination!

Finding Support

If this book has inspired you to make some personal changes, I encourage you to find a support system that can help sustain your intention and reinforce your good choices. For some, this support system simply involves friends and family.

Others benefit from working with a registered holistic nutritionist like me. I offer a range of services that can be reviewed on my website, https://tracyhoule.com/

Together, we will take a close look at your lifestyle, including eating and movement habits. We will identify any nutritional deficiencies or food allergies and sensitivities you may have that may be affecting your health or how you feel in your day-to-day. Working together, we will create an individualized diet plan that fits your needs and interests. To ensure you can succeed in your plan, we will track your progress and support you as you work toward your personal goals. If you are struggling with weight loss or weight gain, have a dietary restriction or chronic illness, or are simply looking for ways to improve your overall health, then a nutrition consultation may be the right choice.

If you prefer to become more informed on your own to be fully empowered to make your food and health choices, I also offer a ten-week course on the connection between food and our moods called The Food & Mood Mindset method, tailored specifically for busy women who want to regain control of their health and their mood. You can learn how to apply the philosophies described in this book as well as a more detailed examination of specific nutrients and their effects on our bodies and minds.

There are additional options for services, ranging from genetic testing for a thorough look at your nutritional needs based on your specific genome to simple meal plans just to get you started.

If you're the type of person to go at it alone, then here are my quick action steps you can start with today. Pick one, three, or all five. It's your choice.

1. Slowly begin to increase your animal protein intake to 0.8 grams to one lb. per pound of body weight and maintain about 130 grams of carbohydrates per day and aim to consume no more than ten to fifteen grams of added sugar per day. This will help to lay the foundation of the natural hunger cues we have lost with overconsumption of processed foods and help to break addiction.

2. Get to know a local farmer. If you live in Canada you can use https://

    regenerationcanada.org if you live in the US
https://www.farmmatch.com

3. Take a quick stock of your cleaning products whether they are household or for your body and see if you can make a few changes to lessen the toxic burden on your health. Use this website to get started. https://www.ewg.org

4. Make time for boredom, it's ok to lounge around your home daily with nothing to do or accomplish.

5. Pick one habit that you wish you did not have and use your newly found growth mindset to replace this outdated habit with a new, more important habit that aligns with your values.

Eventually, our generation will be the ancestors of the past. Whether we aim to or not, we are leaving behind a legacy. I personally want to be part of the generation that took the small steps necessary to create the big change that is inevitably coming, because progress always gets here, eventually.

However you decide to work on your personal health and lifestyle, I wish you all the best as you seek out a new life that aligns your values, your food, your movement, and your most authentic, connected self.

NOTES

Introduction

1. Steve M. Stanley, National Research Council (US) Panel on Effects of Past Global Change on Life, *Effects of Past Global Change on Life* (Washington, DC: National Academies Press, 1995), chap. 14, "Climatic Forcing and the Origin of the Human Genus," https://www.ncbi.nlm.nih.gov/books/NBK231942/.

2. Mario Vaneechoutte et al., "Have We Been Barking up the Wrong Ancestral Tree? Australopithecines Are Probably Not Our Ancestors," Nature Anthropology 2, no. 1 (2024): 10007, https://doi.org/10.35534/natanthropol.2023.10007.

3. Fran Dorey, "Australopithecus bahrelghazali," *Australian Museum*, last updated December 20, 2019, https://australian.museum/learn/science/human-evolution/australopithecus-bahrelghazali/.

4. Briana Pobiner, "Meat-Eating Among the Earliest Humans," *American Scientist*, accessed August 5, 2024, https://www.americanscientist.org/article/meat-eating-among-the-earliest-humans.

5. Ibid.

6. Ibid.

7. Lesley Newson and Peter J. Richerson, "Building Today's World," in *A Story of Us: A New Look at Human Evolution* (Oxford: Oxford University Press, 2021), 144–187, https://doi.org/10.1093/oso/9780190883201.003.0007,

8. Steven Morris, "The 1066 Diet: Normans Passed on Their Love of Pork, Study Suggests," *The Guardian*, July 6, 2020, https://www.theguardian.com/science/2020/jul/06/the-1066-diet-normans-passed-on-their-love-of-pork-study-suggests.

9. James H. O'Keefe, Robert Vogel, Carl J. Lavie, and Loren Cordain, "Achieving Hunter-Gatherer Fitness in the 21st Century: Back to the Future," *The American Journal of Medicine* 123, no. 10 (2010): 1082-1086, https://doi.org/10.1016/j.amjmed.2010.04.026

10. Daniel Lieberman, *The Story of the Human Body: Evolution, Health and Disease* (New York: Vintage, 2014).

1. The Hidden Addiction

1. Loren Cordain, "Cereal Grains: Humanity's Double-Edged Sword," *World Review of Nutrition and Dietetics* 84 (1999): 19-73, https://doi.org/10.1159/000059677.
2. Ibid.
3. Ibid.
4. UNICEF, "Nearly Two in Three Children in Need Were Protected with the Requisite Two Annual High Dose Vitamin A Supplements in 2022," last updated March 2023, https://data.unicef.org/topic/nutrition/vitamin-a-deficiency/.
5. Denise Schatt-Denslow, "Sweet Poison: Exploring the Dangerous Impact of Sugar on Mental Health," *The JEM Foundation*, February 26, 2024, https://thejemfoundation.com/dangerous-impact-of-sugar-on-mental-health.
6. Ibid.
7. Lauren Panoff, "Is Cheese Addictive?" *Healthline*, December 11, 2019, https://www.healthline.com/nutrition/is-cheese-addictive.
8. Keith Bernard Woodford, "Casomorphins and Gliadorphins Have Diverse Systemic Effects Spanning Gut, Brain and Internal Organs," *International Journal of Environmental Research and Public Health* 18, no. 15 (August 2021): https://doi.org/10.3390/ijerph18157911.
9. James Greenblatt, "Food Addiction: The Chemistry of Dairy & Wheat," *Psychiatry Redefined*, January 15, 2021, https://www.psychiatryredefined.org/food-addiction-dairy-and-wheat.
10. Michael Moss, *Salt, Sugar, Fat: How the Food Giants Hooked Us* (New York: Random House Trade Paperbacks, 2014).
11. Nell Boeschenstein, "How the Food Industry Manipulates Taste Buds with 'Salt, Sugar, Fat'," *NPR*, February 26, 2013, https://www.npr.org/sections/thesalt/2013/02/26/172969363/how-the-food-industry-manipulates-taste-buds-with-salt-sugar-fat.
12. Ibid.
13. Moss, *Salt, Sugar, Fat*, p. 10
14. Ibid., p. 99
15. Ibid.
16. Colin Schultz, "Ten Percent of Americans Drink Half the Booze," *Smithsonian Magazine*, September 26, 2014, https://www.smithsonianmag.com/smart-news/ten-percent-americans-drink-half-booze-180952857/.

2. The Problem with Going Meatless

1. The PEW Environment Group, *Big Chicken: Pollution and Industrial Poultry Production in America* (July 27, 2011), https://www.pewtrusts.org/~/media/legacy/uploadedfiles/peg/publications/report/pegbigchickenjuly2011pdf.pdf.

2. Peter Castleberry, "Chicken CAFOs," *Black Warrior Riverkeeper*, accessed August 5, 2024, https://blackwarriorriver.org/cafos/.

3. Chris Kresser, "Why Grass-Fed Trumps Grain-Fed," *ChrisKresser.com*, last modified August 12, 2019, https://chriskresser.com/why-grass-fed-trumps-grain-fed-and-why-you-should-try-it/.

4. Joséphine Gehring et al., "Consumption of Ultra-Processed Foods by Pesco-Vegetarians, Vegetarians, and Vegans: Associations with Duration and Age at Diet Initiation," *Journal of Nutrition* 151, no. 1 (January 4, 2021): 120-131, https://doi.org/10.1093/jn/nxaa196.

5. Lynda W. Powell, *The Influence of Campaign Contributions in State Legislatures: The Effects of Institutions and Politics* (Ann Arbor: University of Michigan Press, 2012), https://doi.org/10.3998/mpub.2454352.

6. Marion Nestle, "Food Industry Lobbyists Running the Dietary Guidelines?" *Food Politics*, February 7, 2018, https://www.foodpolitics.com/2018/02/food-industry-lobbyists-running-the-dietary-guidelines/.

7. Peter Kogut, "Monoculture Farming in Agriculture Industry," *EOS Data Analytics*, October 20, 2020, https://eos.com/blog/monoculture-farming.

8. Global Food Justice Alliance, "Myth Busting Meatless Mondays: Why Meat Is a Powerful Ally for School Nutrition," accessed August 5, 2024, https://www.globalfoodjustice.org/nutrition/meatlessmondaymyths.

3. The Power of Local

1. Drew DeSilver, "What the Data Says About Food Stamps in the U.S.," *PEW Research Center*, July 19, 2023, https://www.pewresearch.org/short-reads/2023/07/19/what-the-data-says-about-food-stamps-in-the-u-s/.

2. Ibid.

3. Zach Conrad et al., "Cardiometabolic Mortality by Supplemental Nutrition Assistance Program Participation and Eligibility in the United States," *American Journal of Public Health* 107, no. 3

(March 2017): 466-474, https://doi.org/10.2105/AJPH.2016.
303608.

4. Mark Hyman, *The Ultramind Solution: Fix Your Broken Brain by Healing Your Body First* (New York: Scribner, 2009).

5. Ibid., p. 3

6. DeSilver, "What the Data Says About Food Stamps in the U.S."

7. Hyman, *The Food Fix*, p. 94.

8. Ibid., p. 95

9. Ibid., p. 327.

4. Environmental Sabotage

1. U.S. Department of Health and Human Services, National Institutes of Health, National Cancer Institute, *Reducing Environmental Cancer Risk: What We Can Do Now*, April 2010, https://deainfo.nci.nih.gov/advisory/pcp/annualreports/pcp08-09rpt/pcp_report_08-09_508.pdf.

2. Ibid, p. 5

3. United States Environmental Protection Agency, "Glyphosate," last updated September 11, 2023, https://www.epa.gov/ingredients-used-pesticide-products/glyphosate.

4. Charles M. Benbrook, "Trends in Glyphosate Herbicide Use in the United States and Globally: Supporting Data." *Environmental Sciences Europe* 28, no. 3 (2016). https://doi.org/10.1186/s12302-016-0070-0.

5. Carmen Costas-Ferreira, Rafael Durán, and Lilian R. F. Faro. "Toxic Effects of Glyphosate on the Nervous System: A Systematic Review." *International Journal of Molecular Sciences* 23, no. 9 (April 21, 2022): 4605. https://doi.org/10.3390/ijms23094605.

6. United States Environmental Protection Agency, "Glyphosate," last updated September 11, 2023, https://www.epa.gov/ingredients-used-pesticide-products/glyphosate.

7. Ibid.

8. Zongzhen Wu, Long Ma, Deqi Su, and Bayindala Xiagedeer, "The Disrupting Effect of Chlormequat Chloride on Growth Hormone Is Associated with Pregnancy," *Toxicology Letters* 395 (2024), https://doi.org/10.1016/j.toxlet.2024.03.004.

9. Endocrine Society, "Impact of EDCs on Metabolism and Obesity," *Endocrine Society*, accessed August 5, 2024, https://www.endocrine.org/topics/edc/what-edcs-are/common-edcs/metabolic.

10. Ibid.

11. The Environmental Working Group (EWG) can be found online at https://ewg.org

12. Elizabeth L. Yu and Jeffrey B. Schwimmer, "Epidemiology of Pediatric Nonalcoholic Fatty Liver Disease," *Clinical Liver Disease* 17, no. 3 (March 2021): 196–199, https://doi.org/10.1002/cld.1027.

13. Children's Health, "Fatty Liver Disease in Children Is on the Rise," accessed August 5, 2024, https://www.childrens.com/health-wellness/fatty-liver-disease-in-children-on-the-rise.

14. Ibid.

15. Nicola Cosentino et al., "Vitamin D and Cardiovascular Disease: Current Evidence and Future Perspectives," *Nutrients* 13, no. 10 (2021): 3603, https://doi.org/10.3390/nu13103603.

16. Gabrielle Lyon, *Forever Strong: A New, Science-Based Strategy for Aging Well* (New York: Atria Books, 2023).

17. Harvard Medical School, "Strength Training Builds More Than Muscles," *Harvard Health Publishing*, January 16, 2024, https://www.health.harvard.edu/staying-healthy/strength-training-builds-more-than-muscles.

18. Ina Shaw and Brandon S. Shaw, "Relationship between Resistance Training and Lipoprotein Profiles in Sedentary Male Smokers," *Cardiovascular Journal of Africa* 19, no. 4 (July-August 2008): 194-197, PMID: 18776961, PMCID: PMC3971764.

19. Ayla Karine Fortunato et al., "Strength Training Session Induces Important Changes on Physiological, Immunological, and Inflammatory Biomarkers," *Journal of Immunology Research*, June 26, 2018, 9675216, https://doi.org/10.1155/2018/9675216.

5. In the Mood

1. Maria C. Giannakourou and Petros S. Taoukis, "Effect of Alternative Preservation Steps and Storage on Vitamin C Stability in Fruit and Vegetable Products: Critical Review and Kinetic Modelling Approaches," *Foods* 10, no. 11 (October 29, 2021): 2630, https://doi.org/10.3390/foods10112630.

2. Center for Disease Control, "Get the Facts: Added Sugars," *CDC Nutrition*, January 5, 2024, https://www.cdc.gov/nutrition/php/data-research/added-sugars.html.

3. Mark Hyman, *The Ultramind Solution: Fix Your Broken Brain by Healing Your Body First* (New York: Scribner, 2009).

4. ibid, p. 56

5. Julia Ross, *The Mood Cure: The 4-Step Program to Rebalance Your Emotional Chemistry and Rediscover Your Natural Sense of Well-Being* (New York: Viking, 2002).

6. Ibid.

7. Ibid.

8. Kaitlin Vogel, "More Young People Are Being Prescribed Antidepressants, Here's Why," *Healthline*, 2024, https://www.health line.com.

9. Laura Ellingson et al., "Changes in Sedentary Time Are Associated with Changes in Mental Wellbeing over 1 Year in Young Adults," *Preventive Medicine Reports* 11 (2018): 274-281, https://doi.org/10.1016/j.pmedr.2018.07.013.

10. Liyuan Jiang et al., "Association of Sedentary Behavior with Anxiety, Depression, and Suicide Ideation in College Students," *Frontiers in Psychiatry* 11 (2020): 1-9, https://doi.org/10.3389/fpsyt.2020.566098.

11. Ellingson, "Changes in Sedentary Time."

12. Carl J. Lavie et al., "Exercise Training and Cardiac Rehabilitation in Primary and Secondary Prevention of Coronary Heart Disease," *Mayo Clinic Proceedings* 84, no. 4 (2009): 373–383, https://doi.org/10.1016/S0025-6196(11)60548-X.

13. Ross, *The Mood Cure*.

6. Reconnect with Our Ancestors

1. Nina Teicholz, *The Big Fat Surprise: Why Butter, Meat, and Cheese Belong in a Healthy Diet* (New York: Simon & Schuster Paperbacks, 2015).

2. Ivan Oransky, "Ancel Keys," *The Lancet* 364, no. 9447 (2004): 1730, https://doi.org/10.1016/S0140-6736(04)17578-8.

3. Teicholz, *The Big Fat Surprise*.

4. Cristin E. Kearns, Laura A. Schmidt, and Stanton A. Glantz, "Sugar Industry and Coronary Heart Disease Research: A Historical Analysis of Internal Industry Documents," *JAMA Internal Medicine* 176, no. 11 (2016): 1680–1685, https://doi.org/10.1001/jamainternmed.2016.5394.

5. Joseph Mercola, *Fat for Fuel: A Revolutionary Diet to Combat Cancer, Boost Brain Power, and Increase Your Energy* (Carlsbad, CA: Hay House Inc., 2017).

6. John H. Cummings and Amanda Engineer, "Denis Burkitt and the Origins of the Dietary Fibre Hypothesis," *Nutrition Research Reviews* 31, no. 1 (2018): 1-15, https://doi.org/10.1017/S0954422417000117.

7. Kok-Yang Tan and Francis Seow-Choen, "Fiber and Colorectal Diseases: Separating Fact from Fiction," *World Journal of Gastroenterology* 13, no. 31 (August 21, 2007): 4161-4167, https://doi.org/10.3748/wjg.v13.i31.4161.

8. W. A. Price, *Nutrition and Physical Degeneration* (New York: Paul B. Hoeber, Inc., 1939).

9. Sally Fallon and Mary G. Enig, "Guts and Grease: The Diets of Native Americans," *Weston A. Price,* accessed August 5, 2024, https://www.westonaprice.org/health-topics/traditional-diets/guts-and-grease-the-diet-of-native-americans/.

7. You Are What You Eat

1. Raffael Heiss, Brigitte Naderer, and Jörg Matthes, "Healthwashing in High-Sugar Food Advertising: The Effect of Prior Information on Healthwashing Perceptions in Austria," *Health Promotion International* 36, no. 4 (August 2021): 1029–1038, published December 8, 2020, https://doi.org/10.1093/heapro/daaa086.

2. Food and Drug Administration, "Use of the Term Natural on Food Labeling," May 2016, https://www.fda.gov/food/food-labeling-nutrition/use-term-natural-food-labeling.

3. Linda Verrill et al., "Vitamin-Fortified Snack Food May Lead Consumers to Make Poor Dietary Decisions," *Journal of the Academy of Nutrition and Dietetics* 117, no. 3 (2017): 376-385, https://doi.org/10.1016/j.jand.2016.10.008, https://www.sciencedirect.com/science/article/pii/S2212267216312151.

4. Linda Verrill et al., "Vitamin-Fortified Snack Food May Lead Consumers to Make Poor Dietary Decisions," *Journal of the Academy of Nutrition and Dietetics*, published December 1, 2016, https://doi.org/10.1016/j.jand.2016.10.008.

5. Ibid.

6. Verrill et al., "Vitamin-Fortified Snack Food."

7. Gastón Ares et al., "Health-Washing of Ultraprocessed Products on Instagram: Prevalence and Strategies in an Emerging Market," *Journal of Nutrition Education and Behavior* 55, no. 11 (2023): 815–822, https://doi.org/10.1016/j.jneb.2023.09.001.

8. Raffael Heiss, Brigitte Naderer, and Jörg Matthes, "Healthwashing in High-Sugar Food Advertising: The Effect of Prior Information on Healthwashing Perceptions in Austria," Health Promotion International 36, no. 4 (August 2021): 1029–1038, https://doi.org/10.1093/heapro/daaa086.

9. Mark Carney, *Value(s): Climate, Credit, Covid and How We Focus on What Matters* (London: William Collins, 2021).

10. Mark Carney, *Value(s): Building a Better World for All* (New York: PublicAffairs, 2021).

8. The Case for Boredom

1. Artem Dogtiev, "Push Notifications Statistics," Business of Apps, May 2, 2024, https://www.businessofapps.com/marketplace/push-notifications/research/push-notifications-statistics/.

2. Beata Mostafavi, "Study: Average Teen Received More Than 200 App Notifications a Day," Michigan Medicine Health Lab, September 26, 2023, https://www.michiganmedicine.org/health-lab/study-average-teen-received-more-200-app-notifications-day.

3. Timothy D. Wilson et al., "Just Think: The Challenges of the Disengaged Mind," Science 345 (2014): 75-77, https://doi.org/10.1126/science.1250830.

4. David M. Ndetei, Paul Nyamai, and Vincent Mutiso, "Boredom-Understanding the Emotion and Its Impact on Our Lives: An African Perspective," Frontiers in Sociology 8 (June 29, 2023), https://doi.org/10.3389/fsoc.2023.1213190.

5. Sandi Mann, *The Science of Boredom: The Upside (and Downside) of Downtime* (London: Robinson, 2018).

6. Elkhonon Goldberg, *The New Executive Brain: Frontal Lobes in a Complex World* (New York: Oxford University Press, 2009).

7. "5 Benefits of Boredom," *Psychology Today*, April 4, 2020, www.psychologytoday.com/us/blog/science-choice/202004/5-benefits-boredom. Accessed May 31, 2024.

8. "Let Your Children Be Bored," *Psychology Today*, February 23, 2024, www.psychologytoday.com/us/blog/decade-of-childhood/202402/let-your-children-be-bored. Accessed May 31, 2024.

9. Matthew Walker, *Why We Sleep* (New York: Penguin Books, 2018).

10. "Brain May Flush Out Toxins During Sleep," *National Institutes of Health (NIH)*, August 6, 2015, www.nih.gov/news-events/news-releases/brain-may-flush-out-toxins-during-sleep. Accessed May 31, 2024.

11. Alex Roddie, "Boredom Is Impossible When Immersed in Nature," Alex Roddie, June 2, 2018, https://www.alexroddie.com/2018/06/boredom-is-impossible-when-immersed-in-nature/.

9. Collective Food

1. "The 5 Steps from Food Security to Famine," *World Food Programme*, March 18, 2024, https://www.wfp.org/stories/5-steps-food-security-famine.

2. Ibid.

3. World Food Program USA, https://www.wfpusa.org/, Accessed August 5, 2024.

4. *Global Nutrition Report: Stronger Commitments for Greater Action* (Bristol, UK: Development Initiatives, 2022), https://globalnutritionreport.org/reports/2020-global-nutrition-report/introduction-towards-global-nutrition-equity/.

5. Ibid.

6. "Spotlight 4.2: The High Cost of Nutritious Foods in Poorer Countries," in *Global Nutrition Report: Stronger Commitments for Greater Action* (Bristol, UK: Development Initiatives, 2022).

7. "Spotlight 4.1: Towards a More Diverse Agri-Food System – Beyond Staple Grains," in *Global Nutrition Report: Stronger Commitments for Greater Action* (Bristol, UK: Development Initiatives, 2022).

8. Ibid.

9. "The Global Food Crisis, Explained," YouTube video, 19:45, uploaded by The Economist, July 19, 2022, www.youtube.com/watch?v=oQWaw5S4b3I.

10. Gouri Sankar Bhunia and Anil Kashyap, "Land Reclamation and Restoration Strategies for Sustainable Development," in *Modern Cartography Series*, 2021, https://www.sciencedirect.com/topics/earth-and-planetary-sciences/land-degradation.

11. Ibid.

12. Savory Institute, "What is Holistic Management?" January 29, 2020, https://savory.global/what-is-holistic-management/.

13. Ibid.

14. Ibid.

15. "A Framework for Managing Complexity," *Savory Institute*, accessed August 5, 2024, https://savory.global/holistic-management/.

16. The Savory Institute, The Foundations of Holistic Management, eBook (2019).

10. All in Your Head

1. Carol S. Dweck, *Mindset* (New York: Ballantine Books, 2008).

2. Ibid., p. 94-98.

3. "No Level of Alcohol Consumption Is Safe for Our Health," *World Health Organization*, January 4, 2023, https://www.who.int/europe/news/item/04-01-2023-no-level-of-alcohol-consumption-is-safe-for-our-health (accessed June 12, 2024).

BIBLIOGRAPHY

"5 Benefits of Boredom." *Psychology Today*. April 4, 2020. www.psychologytoday.com/us/blog/science-choice/202004/5-benefits-boredom. Accessed May 31, 2024.

"A Framework for Managing Complexity." *Savory Institute*. Accessed August 5, 2024. https://savory.global/holistic-management/.

"Brain May Flush Out Toxins During Sleep." *National Institutes of Health (NIH)*. August 6, 2015. www.nih.gov/news-events/news-releases/brain-may-flush-out-toxins-during-sleep. Accessed May 31, 2024.

"Let Your Children Be Bored." *Psychology Today*. February 23, 2024. www.psychologytoday.com/us/blog/decade-of-childhood/202402/let-your-children-be-bored. Accessed May 31, 2024.

"Spotlight 4.1: Towards a More Diverse Agri-Food System – Beyond Staple Grains." In *Global Nutrition Report: Stronger Commitments for Greater Action*. Bristol, UK: Development Initiatives, 2022.

"Spotlight 4.2: The High Cost of Nutritious Foods in Poorer Countries." In *Global Nutrition Report: Stronger Commitments for Greater Action*. Bristol, UK: Development Initiatives, 2022.

"The 5 Steps from Food Security to Famine." *World Food Programme*. March 18, 2024. https://www.wfp.org/stories/5-steps-food-security-famine.

"The Global Food Crisis, Explained." YouTube video, 19:45. Uploaded by *The Economist*. July 19, 2022. www.youtube.com/watch?v=oQWaw5S4b3I.

Benbrook, Charles M. "Trends in Glyphosate Herbicide Use in the United States and Globally: Supporting Data." *Environmental Sciences Europe* 28, no. 3 (2016). https://doi.org/10.1186/s12302-016-0070-0.

Bhunia, Gouri Sankar and Anil Kashyap. "Land Reclamation and Restoration Strategies for Sustainable Development." In *Modern Cartography Series*. 2021. https://www.sciencedirect.com/topics/earth-and-planetary-sciences/land-degradation.

Boeschenstein, Nell. "How the Food Industry Manipulates Taste Buds with 'Salt, Sugar, Fat'." *NPR*. February 26, 2013. https://www.npr.

org/sections/thesalt/2013/02/26/172969363/how-the-food-indus try-manipulates-taste-buds-with-salt-sugar-fat.

Carney, Mark. *Value(s): Building a Better World for All.* New York: PublicAffairs, 2021.

Carney, Mark. *Value(s): Climate, Credit, Covid and How We Focus on What Matters.* London: William Collins, 2021.

Castleberry, Peter. "Chicken CAFOs." *Black Warrior Riverkeeper.* Accessed August 5, 2024. https://blackwarriorriver.org/cafos/.

Center for Disease Control. "Get the Facts: Added Sugars." *CDC Nutrition.* January 5, 2024. https://www.cdc.gov/nutrition/php/ data-research/added-sugars.html.

Conrad, Zach et al. "Cardiometabolic Mortality by Supplemental Nutrition Assistance Program Participation and Eligibility in the United States." *American Journal of Public Health* 107, no. 3 (March 2017): 466-474. https://doi.org/10.2105/AJPH.2016. 303608.

Cordain, Loren. "Cereal Grains: Humanity's Double-Edged Sword." *World Review of Nutrition and Dietetics* 84 (1999): 19-73. https:// doi.org/10.1159/000059677.

Costas-Ferreira, Carmen, Rafael Durán, and Lilian R. F. Faro. "Toxic Effects of Glyphosate on the Nervous System: A Systematic Review." *International Journal of Molecular Sciences* 23, no. 9 (April 21, 2022): 4605. https://doi.org/10.3390/ijms23094605.

Dorey, Fran. "Australopithecus bahrelghazali." *Australian Museum.* Last updated December 20, 2019. https://australian.museum/ learn/science/human-evolution/australopithecus-bahrelghazali/.

Dogtiev, Artem. "Push Notifications Statistics." *Business of Apps.* May 2, 2024. https://www.businessofapps.com/marketplace/push-notifi cations/research/push-notifications-statistics/.

Drew DeSilver. "What the Data Says About Food Stamps in the U.S." *PEW Research Center.* July 19, 2023. https://www.pewresearch. org/short-reads/2023/07/19/what-the-data-says-about-food- stamps-in-the-u-s/.

Dweck, Carol S. *Mindset.* New York: Ballantine Books, 2008.

Endocrine Society. "Impact of EDCs on Metabolism and Obesity." *Endocrine Society.* Accessed August 5, 2024. https://www. endocrine.org/topics/edc/what-edcs-are/common-edcs/metabolic.

Fallon, Sally and Mary G. Enig. "Guts and Grease: The Diets of Native Americans." *Weston A. Price.* Accessed August 5, 2024. https:// www.westonaprice.org/health-topics/traditional-diets/guts-and- grease-the-diet-of-native-americans/.

Food and Drug Administration. "Use of the Term Natural on Food Labeling." May 2016. https://www.fda.gov/food/food-labeling-nutrition/use-term-natural-food-labeling.

Fortunato, Ayla Karine et al. "Strength Training Session Induces Important Changes on Physiological, Immunological, and Inflammatory Biomarkers." *Journal of Immunology Research.* June 26, 2018. 9675216. https://doi.org/10.1155/2018/9675216.

Gehring, Joséphine et al. "Consumption of Ultra-Processed Foods by Pesco-Vegetarians, Vegetarians, and Vegans: Associations with Duration and Age at Diet Initiation." *Journal of Nutrition* 151, no. 1 (January 4, 2021): 120-131. https://doi.org/10.1093/jn/nxaa196.

Giannakourou, Maria C. and Petros S. Taoukis. "Effect of Alternative Preservation Steps and Storage on Vitamin C Stability in Fruit and Vegetable Products: Critical Review and Kinetic Modelling Approaches." *Foods* 10, no. 11 (October 29, 2021): 2630. https://doi.org/10.3390/foods10112630.

Global Nutrition Report. *Stronger Commitments for Greater Action.* Bristol, UK: Development Initiatives, 2022. https://globalnutrition report.org/reports/2020-global-nutrition-report/introduction-towards-global-nutrition-equity/.

Goldberg, Elkhonon. *The New Executive Brain: Frontal Lobes in a Complex World.* New York: Oxford University Press, 2009.

Greenblatt, James. "Food Addiction: The Chemistry of Dairy & Wheat." *Psychiatry Redefined.* January 15, 2021. https://www.psychiatryredefined.org/food-addiction-dairy-and-wheat.

Harvard Medical School. "Strength Training Builds More Than Muscles." *Harvard Health Publishing.* January 16, 2024. https://www.health.harvard.edu/staying-healthy/strength-training-builds-more-than-muscles.

Heiss, Raffael, Brigitte Naderer, and Jörg Matthes. "Healthwashing in High-Sugar Food Advertising: The Effect of Prior Information on Healthwashing Perceptions in Austria." *Health Promotion International* 36, no. 4 (August 2021): 1029–1038. Published December 8, 2020. https://doi.org/10.1093/heapro/daaa086.

Houghtaling, Bailey et al. "A Rapid Review of Stocking and Marketing Practices Used to Sell Sugar-Sweetened Beverages in U.S. Food Stores." *Obesity Reviews* 22, no. 4 (April 2021): e13179. Published online December 16, 2020. https://doi.org/10.1111/obr.13179.

Hyman, Mark. *The Ultramind Solution: Fix Your Broken Brain by Healing Your Body First.* New York: Scribner, 2009.

Hyman, Mark. *The Food Fix.* New York: Scribner, 2009.

Jiang, Liyuan et al. "Association of Sedentary Behavior with Anxiety, Depression, and Suicide Ideation in College Students." *Frontiers in Psychiatry* 11 (2020): 1-9. https://doi.org/10.3389/fpsyt.2020.566098.

Kim, Hae Dun et al. "Sleep-Inducing Effect of Lettuce (Lactuca sativa) Varieties on Pentobarbital-Induced Sleep." *Food Science and Biotechnology* 26, no. 3 (2017): 807–814. Published online May 29, 2017. https://doi.org/10.1007/s10068-017-0107-1.

Kogut, Peter. "Monoculture Farming in Agriculture Industry." *EOS Data Analytics*. October 20, 2020. https://eos.com/blog/monoculture-farming.

Lavie, Carl J. et al. "Exercise Training and Cardiac Rehabilitation in Primary and Secondary Prevention of Coronary Heart Disease." *Mayo Clinic Proceedings* 84, no. 4 (2009): 373–383. https://doi.org/10.1016/S0025-6196(11)60548-X.

Lieberman, Daniel. *The Story of the Human Body: Evolution, Health and Disease*. New York: Vintage, 2014.

Lyon, Gabrielle. *Forever Strong: A New, Science-Based Strategy for Aging Well*. New York: Atria Books, 2023.

Mann, Sandi. *The Science of Boredom: The Upside (and Downside) of Downtime*. London: Robinson, 2018.

Mercola, Joseph. *Fat for Fuel: A Revolutionary Diet to Combat Cancer, Boost Brain Power, and Increase Your Energy*. Carlsbad, CA: Hay House Inc., 2017.

Michael Moss. *Salt, Sugar, Fat: How the Food Giants Hooked Us*. New York: Random House Trade Paperbacks, 2014.

Morris, Steven. "The 1066 Diet: Normans Passed on Their Love of Pork, Study Suggests." *The Guardian*. July 6, 2020. https://www.theguardian.com/science/2020/jul/06/the-1066-diet-normans-passed-on-their-love-of-pork-study-suggests.

Nestle, Marion. "Food Industry Lobbyists Running the Dietary Guidelines?" *Food Politics*. February 7, 2018. https://www.foodpolitics.com/2018/02/food-industry-lobbyists-running-the-dietary-guidelines/.

Newson, Lesley and Peter J. Richerson. "Building Today's World." In *A Story of Us: A New Look at Human Evolution*. Oxford: Oxford University Press, 2021. 144–187. https://doi.org/10.1093/oso/9780190883201.003.0007.

Ndetei, David M., Paul Nyamai, and Vincent Mutiso. "Boredom-Understanding the Emotion and Its Impact on Our Lives: An

African Perspective." *Frontiers in Sociology* 8 (June 29, 2023). https://doi.org/10.3389/fsoc.2023.1213190.

O'Keefe, James H., Robert Vogel, Carl J. Lavie, and Loren Cordain. "Achieving Hunter-Gatherer Fitness in the 21st Century: Back to the Future." *The American Journal of Medicine* 123, no. 10 (2010): 1082-1086. https://doi.org/10.1016/j.amjmed.2010.04.026.

Panoff, Lauren. "Is Cheese Addictive?" *Healthline.* December 11, 2019. https://www.healthline.com/nutrition/is-cheese-addictive.

Pobiner, Briana. "Meat-Eating Among the Earliest Humans." *American Scientist.* Accessed August 5, 2024. https://www.americanscientist.org/article/meat-eating-among-the-earliest-humans.

Price, W. A. *Nutrition and Physical Degeneration.* New York: Paul B. Hoeber, Inc., 1939.

Roddie, Alex. "Boredom Is Impossible When Immersed in Nature." *Alex Roddie.* June 2, 2018. https://www.alexroddie.com/2018/06/boredom-is-impossible-when-immersed-in-nature/.

Ross, Julia. *The Mood Cure: The 4-Step Program to Rebalance Your Emotional Chemistry and Rediscover Your Natural Sense of Well-Being.* New York: Viking, 2002.

Savory Institute. "What is Holistic Management?" January 29, 2020. https://savory.global/what-is-holistic-management/.

Savory Institute. *The Foundations of Holistic Management.* eBook (2019).

Schatt-Denslow, Denise. "Sweet Poison: Exploring the Dangerous Impact of Sugar on Mental Health." *The JEM Foundation.* February 26, 2024. https://thejemfoundation.com/dangerous-impact-of-sugar-on-mental-health.

Schultz, Colin. "Ten Percent of Americans Drink Half the Booze." *Smithsonian Magazine.* September 26, 2014. https://www.smithsonianmag.com/smart-news/ten-percent-americans-drink-half-booze-180952857/.

Stanley, Steve M. *National Research Council (US) Panel on Effects of Past Global Change on Life. Effects of Past Global Change on Life* (Washington, DC: National Academies Press, 1995). Chap. 14, "Climatic Forcing and the Origin of the Human Genus." https://www.ncbi.nlm.nih.gov/books/NBK231942/.

Teicholz, Nina. *The Big Fat Surprise: Why Butter, Meat, and Cheese Belong in a Healthy Diet.* New York: Simon & Schuster Paperbacks, 2015.

Timothy D. Wilson et al. "Just Think: The Challenges of the Disengaged Mind." *Science* 345 (2014): 75-77. https://doi.org/10.1126/science.1250830.

UNICEF. "Nearly Two in Three Children in Need Were Protected with the Requisite Two Annual High Dose Vitamin A Supplements in 2022." Last updated March 2023. https://data.unicef.org/topic/nutrition/vitamin-a-deficiency/.

United States Environmental Protection Agency. "Glyphosate." Last updated September 11, 2023. https://www.epa.gov/ingredients-used-pesticide-products/glyphosate.

Verrill, Linda et al. "Vitamin-Fortified Snack Food May Lead Consumers to Make Poor Dietary Decisions." *Journal of the Academy of Nutrition and Dietetics* 117, no. 3 (2017): 376-385. https://doi.org/10.1016/j.jand.2016.10.008.   https://www.sciencedirect.com/science/article/pii/S2212267216312151.

Walker, Matthew. *Why We Sleep.* New York: Penguin Books, 2018.

Woodford, Keith Bernard. "Casomorphins and Gliadorphins Have Diverse Systemic Effects Spanning Gut, Brain and Internal Organs." *International Journal of Environmental Research and Public Health* 18, no. 15 (August 2021): https://doi.org/10.3390/ijerph18157911.

Wu, Zongzhen, Long Ma, Deqi Su, and Bayindala Xiagedeer. "The Disrupting Effect of Chlormequat Chloride on Growth Hormone Is Associated with Pregnancy." *Toxicology Letters* 395 (2024). https://doi.org/10.1016/j.toxlet.2024.03.004.

ABOUT THE AUTHOR

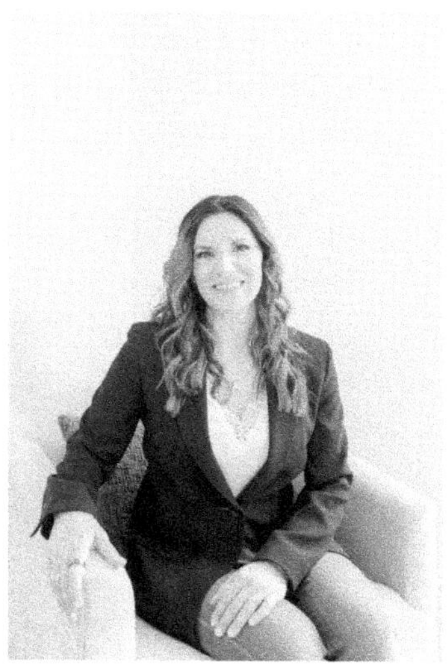

Tracy Houle, RHN, is an esteemed professional in the health and wellness industry, boasting over ten years of dedicated experience. Her passion for holistic health and nutrition has established her as a trusted authority on achieving true well-being through balanced living.

As the visionary founder of tracyhoule.com, Tracy has created a thriving platform where she offers personalized health coaching and meticulously designed wellness programs. Her commitment to empowering individuals to take control of their health journeys is evident in her hands-on approach and the tailored strategies she develops for each client. This personalized methodology has proven incredibly effective, evidenced by the countless clients who have achieved and surpassed their health and fitness goals under her guidance.

Tracy's achievements go beyond individual success stories; she is also a published author, contributing valuable knowledge and insights to the broader conversation on health and wellness. Her articles serve as a testament to her breadth of knowledge and dedication to spreading awareness about nutrition, fitness, and the importance of a holistic lifestyle.

With a professional background deeply rooted in holistic health practices, Tracy Houle has distinguished herself as an expert in nutrition and the mind body connection. Her comprehensive approach ensures that her clients not only reach their immediate health goals but also acquire the tools and knowledge necessary for lifelong wellness. Tracy's passion for health is characterized by her unwavering dedication to helping others discover the joy and fulfillment that comes from living a healthy, balanced life.

Learn more about Tracy at https://tracyhoule.com

Or contact her at info@tracyhoule.com

ACKNOWLEDGMENTS

I would like to extend my heartfelt gratitude to Amanda, Emily, and Laura at Page & Podium for their invaluable support in the journey of writing my first book. Your expertise, guidance, and encouragement have made this experience not only possible but truly enjoyable. From brainstorming ideas to refining the final manuscript, your team's dedication has been instrumental in bringing my vision to life. Thank you for being such a wonderful partner in this creative endeavour—I couldn't have done it without you!

I also want to take a moment to express my deepest thanks to my incredible husband, Jason, and our amazing kids, Dante, Sofia, and Luca. You are my constant inspiration in both life and health, and your unwavering support has grounded me in ways I can't fully express. Jason, your encouragement reminds me that dreams are worth pursuing, while Dante, Sofia, and Luca, your laughter and love fuel my passion every day. Together, you keep me motivated to chase after my goals, and for that, I am eternally grateful. Thank you for being my greatest cheerleaders and for believing in me even when I doubted myself. I love you all dearly!

PRAISE FOR TRACY HOULE, RHN

The moment we met Tracy our lives were forever changed! Her dedication and passion for a healthier lifestyle and healthy living is inspiring. Tracy is extremely knowledgeable about nutrition and her meal plans are individualized, easy-to-follow, and most importantly, delicious! She truly takes the time to get to know her clients and supports them to achieve their goals. Tracy gives us hope for a better future, provides a path to follow, and acts as a guide along the journey. Thank you for always going above and beyond!

JENNY

I'm so thankful I found Tracy Houle; her knowledge, care, and compassion are impeccable. My sessions with Tracy provided me with an action plan that has been remarkable for my overall health and well-being. Thank you, Tracy, for the accountability I needed to continue on my path of health and longevity.

MICHELLE L.

Honestly, all I can say is that your positive attitude, your kindness, and reasonable expectations makes this program pleasant and easy to follow and successful. After working with other professionals, Tracy is, by far, the most knowledgeable, kind, reasonable, professional and caring coach. You actually want to help your clients to achieve their goals and you are very reasonable and understanding of all circumstances.

SANDRA

I notice right away now that I am not eating healthy because I am moody and have less control of my emotions. It has really brought awareness to my reactions and my eating habits and how closely those two are linked. Overall the program was amazing. I feel better and have a more positive outlook. I was surprised how much the food portion affected the mindset and vice versa. This program is amazing and is so needed for us busy mamas.

MELISSA

Working with Tracy definitely changed my way of looking at eating certain foods. As much as I love food and sugary snacks, I learned how much sugar has an impact on my body and mind. It really opened up my eyes to the damage I was doing internally. Thank you Tracy for your inspiration and insights on my food choices.

ERIKA